Parent's Quick Start Guide to Autism

Parent's Quick Start Guide to Autism provides parents and caregivers with an immediate overview of autism spectrum disorder (ASD) and the steps they can take to support and encourage their child.

Each chapter is packed with detailed and helpful information, covering what to do at home and at school, how to avoid common mistakes, and how (and when) to seek professional help. Summary and resource sections at the end of each chapter give quick guidance to busy readers. Topics include occupational therapy (OT), applied behavior analysis (ABA), cognitive behavioral therapy (CBT), interventions, and more.

Offering straightforward, easy to understand, and evidence-based information, this book is a go-to resource for caregivers parenting a child with autism.

Noelle Balsamo is Assistant Professor of Special Education at Florida Gulf Coast University, Ft. Myers, where she specializes in autism and related disabilities, applied behavior analysis, and parent education.

James W. Forgan is Associate Professor of Special Education at Florida Atlantic University, Jupiter, where he prepares teachers to teach kids with autism and related disabilities.

Parent's Quick Start Guide to Autism

Noelle Balsamo and James W. Forgan

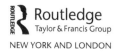

Routledge
Taylor & Francis Group

NEW YORK AND LONDON

Cover image: © Getty Images

First published 2022
by Routledge
605 Third Avenue, New York, NY 10158

and by Routledge
4 Park Square, Milton Park, Abingdon, Oxon, OX14 4RN

Routledge is an imprint of the Taylor & Francis Group, an informa business

Library of Congress Cataloging-in-Publication Data
Names: Balsamo, Noelle, author. | Forgan, James W., author.
Title: Parent's quick start guide to autism / Noelle Balsamo, James W. Forgan.
Description: New York, NY : Routledge, 2022. | Includes bibliographical references. |
Identifiers: LCCN 2021059419 (print) | LCCN 2021059420 (ebook) |
ISBN 9781032259826 (paperback) | ISBN 9781003285953 (ebook)
Subjects: LCSH: Autistic children--Care. | Parents of autistic children. | Parenting. | Autism in children--Treatment.
Classification: LCC RJ506.A9 B253 2022 (print) | LCC RJ506.A9 (ebook) | DDC 618.92/85882--dc23/eng/20211208
LC record available at https://lccn.loc.gov/2021059419
LC ebook record available at https://lccn.loc.gov/2021059420

ISBN: 978-1-032-25982-6 (pbk)
ISBN: 978-1-003-28595-3 (ebk)

DOI: 10.4324/9781003285953

Typeset in Palatino
by Deanta Global Publishing Services, Chennai, India

With gratitude and admiration, Noelle dedicates this book to her daughter, "you are meant for great things in this world." James dedicates this book to his understanding and supportive family.

Contents

Illustrations

Figure

Tables

Boxes

Acknowledgments

Projects like this require the work of many individuals and we'd like to thank our editor Misha Kidd for her expertise as well as the contributions of parents and professionals including Shelly Hedge, Daniely Lins da Silva, Kamal Smith, Toby Honsberger, Ed.D., Cathleen Blair, Raj Shekhat, M.D., Judith Aronson-Ramos, M.D., and Emily Forgan. Thank you all for sharing your hearts and for your tireless work to help families and children.

Introduction

Autism is something you have likely heard about on the news, read about on the internet, and seen portrayed on television or in the movies. But now, you have a loved one with the diagnosis and suddenly autism is real, unfamiliar, and personal. It may suddenly feel like autism is a mystery that you alone have to solve. We assure you this is not the case and that is why we are thrilled you found our book!

An autism diagnosis comes with both unique challenges and unique gifts. It presents an opportunity to gain better insight about your loved one and your relationship with them. From this diagnosis, you have learned that your child is "neurologically" wired differently. This new perspective might shed some light on the social, communication, and behavior differences you may have been questioning for some time. With this diagnosis in hand, you can now seek to better understand your child's differences and learn how to embrace and support the best aspects of them.

That is not to deny the challenging aspects of autism that you and your child may have been struggling through on your own. These challenges are real, and your best parenting strategies may be falling short. Not because you are doing it wrong, but because your child is "hard-wired" to learn differently. Children with autism do not learn to communicate better without effective intervention. Problem behaviors do not go away, but only

DOI: 10.4324/9781003285953-1

get worse without effective intervention. Strengths and talents do not lead to meaningful outcomes without effective teachers and informed advocates.

Now that autism is personal to your life and a known part of who your child is, it is time to position yourself to act on this awareness. You are your child's best teacher and advocate, but you do not need to do this alone.

Embarking on This New Journey

An autism diagnosis may require you to shift gears on how you parent your child and who you trust to help. This may not be a quick or easy journey, but it is a rewarding one with many small successes (words spoken, eyes connected, smiles shared) and exciting achievements to look forward to (goals met, relationships strengthened, independence increased).

Wherever you are on this journey, we encourage you to take a moment to remind yourself and your child that the love and perseverance that carried you to this point will help you face any unexpected challenges you may encounter together from here. Use your words and actions to assure your child that you will always strive to understand and learn from them. You are willing to do whatever it takes and have what it takes to do it.

Let Us Help!

Understanding your child from this new perspective may feel confusing and overwhelming at first. The decisions you make now will greatly determine your child's progress, as early intervention is key. It is understandable that you want to act fast. So, we take you straight to and quickly through the most up-to-date autism research to help you know what to do, why you should do it, and how to get started quickly.

Our goal is to empower you to do what is most helpful for your child and to help you avoid common mistakes parents make as they embark on this journey to guide their sons and daughters from childhood to adulthood. As professionals, we believe helping your child with autism takes:

- ◆ Knowledge about their unique strengths and deficits
- ◆ Choosing evidence-based practices
- ◆ Enlisting the support of trusted professionals (health care, educators, therapists)
- ◆ Maintaining confidence in your child, yourself, and the process
- ◆ Hard work by you and your child

Some of the strategies discussed here, you can do on your own. Others necessitate professional support to protect your child's health and safety and to safeguard your quality time together. We will help you know the difference and help get you connected with a trusted team of support along the way.

Navigating This Resource

Since you are at your own unique stage in this journey, you might need to simply turn to the chapter that is most important to you now. Are there challenging behaviors or routines that interfere with daily life? Are you having trouble knowing how to support your child at school?

Does your child need a specific therapy, but you do not understand why? Here's how we recommend you proceed with this resource:

- ◆ Read the chapter(s) that are most important to you now
- ◆ Prioritize the evidence-based intervention(s) we discuss here based on the safety and well-being of your child and family
- ◆ Identify qualified professionals described here to help you start and stay on the right track
- ◆ Connect or reconnect with trusted social supports (family members, parent groups, advocacy groups, faith-based groups, etc.)
- ◆ Stick to the science and your instincts

A Message from the Authors

As a previous school teacher and now a university professor and author, I am grateful to my students and peers with autism for enlightening me on how they learn best, so I can be a better teacher and ally on their behalf here. I am also grateful for the knowledgeable and concerned professionals that diagnosed my own daughter with autism, allowing me to learn from her and them how to be a better parent and advocate for her and, in turn, provide a more compassionate resource for you on this shared journey. I have benefited from and contributed to the science that informs us on best practices for promoting the independence and well-being of our loved ones and shields us from the misguided practices that don't. It is a privilege to have the opportunity to share my accumulated knowledge and experiences with you in this book.

Dr. Noelle Balsamo

If you are a person of faith, I'd like encourage you with a song. Hillsong United is a contemporary Christian music group and Chris Davenport is a lead singer. Chris wrote the song "Another in the Fire" as his son was given an autism diagnosis. This song strengthened his faith and I hope it strengthens yours too. You can listen to his story at: https://youtu.be/6xrE-JMAfMY.

Dr. James Forgan

We thank you for bringing our book along with you on this journey!

1

Autism

Autism Explained

Autism spectrum disorder (ASD), autism for short, is a lifelong neurodevelopmental disorder that shows up in difficulty with social communication and social interaction along with restricted or repetitive patterns of behavior, interests, or actions. Common autism characteristics include but are not limited to:

♦ Poor, inconsistent, or unusual eye contact
♦ Delayed speech and/or difficulty communicating wants and needs
♦ Immediate or delayed "echoing" of what was heard
♦ Difficulty engaging in two-way conversations
♦ Difficulty starting or maintaining play with others
♦ Difficulty taking turns
♦ Difficulty understanding others' feelings or facial expressions
♦ Difficulty using or understanding gestures (e.g., pointing)
♦ Sensory sensitivities (e.g., avoiding or seeking)
♦ Repetitive auditory (e.g., nonfunctional sounds) and/or motor behaviors (e.g., rocking, hand flapping, spinning objects)
♦ Having an unusual fixation on a specific topic (e.g., trains, horses, Pokémon, dinosaurs, certain numbers or letters, anime, etc.)

DOI: 10.4324/9781003285953-2

- ◆ Difficulty adjusting to change in routines
- ◆ Difficulty with transitions, especially from preferred activities to less preferred ones
- ◆ Difficulty following multi-step directions
- ◆ Might not consistently respond to name
- ◆ Problem behaviors (e.g., aggression towards self or others, frequent tantrums, frequent noncompliance during routine tasks)

Diagnosing Autism

We assume by you reading this book that your child has an autism spectrum disorder diagnosis, henceforth referred to as autism. If not, it's important to get a reliable diagnosis. Many parents receive what is called a "medical diagnosis" that comes from an experienced:

- ◆ Psychiatrist
- ◆ Psychologist/school psychologist
- ◆ Neurologist
- ◆ Developmental pediatrician

You want to work with a professional or team of professionals who uses a thorough diagnostic approach involving interaction with your child and discussion with you and others who know your child well. Most professionals diagnose using a combination of interviewing, rating scales, direct observation, and testing with your child.

The American Psychiatric Association publishes the *Diagnostic and Statistical Manual of Mental Disorders* (2013, DSM-5), which holds the complete diagnostic criteria for ASD. There you will see that autism is diagnosed based on common characteristics seen across two specific areas: Social Communication and Restrictive and Repetitive Behaviors (examples of each are provided in the list in the section above called "Autism Explained"). A child must show characteristics in both areas to be reliably diagnosed.

In general, five criteria should be met to diagnose autism. First, the child must demonstrate persistent deficits in social communication and social interaction across settings. Second, the child must display restricted, repetitive patterns of behavior, interests, or activities, currently or by history. Third, the child's symptoms must have been present in the early developmental period. Fourth, there must be evidence of clinically significant impairment in social, academic, or occupational functioning. Fifth, the symptoms must not be caused by another mental or physical condition.

The DSM-5 also describes a child's autism diagnosis by the level of support they are likely to need. These levels are:

- ◆ Requiring support (mild)
- ◆ Requiring substantial support (moderate)
- ◆ Requiring very substantial support (severe)

Some parents learn their child has autism through the public school system's evaluation process and this is considered an "educational eligibility" for services rather than a true autism diagnosis. Schools are not in the business of diagnosing children with disorders but rather providing what is called a "free appropriate public education" for any child with a disability. Thus, if the school staff tell you your child meets eligibility for services under the category of autism, that simply provides school services. You might still need a "medical diagnosis" of autism from a medical professional to receive services, such as private speech or applied behavior analysis (ABA) therapies, from providers on your health insurance plan.

What the Research Reports

Autism is a lifelong disorder that can be diagnosed as early as two years old (Lord, 1995). Catherine Lord studied thirty two-year-old children for possible autism and found that young children can be reliably diagnosed. She posed the question, "What are autistic children like at two years of age?" and afterwards answered it. They differed from other children in having a lack of initiative in seeking visual attention, a lack of response to voice, difficulty understanding gesture, unusual use of others' bodies, unusual hand and finger mannerisms, and unusual sensory behaviors. She reported, "Deficits in two areas, directing others' attention and attention to voice were the clearest discriminators of autism in these young children on an individual as well as group basis" (p. 1380).

Pediatricians often begin screening children for autism warning signs as early as one year of age, beginning with a family history to determine if any family members, especially a sibling, has been diagnosed with autism. Johnson and Myers (2007) summarized that,

> Some of the very early signs reported by several investigators include extremes of temperament and behavior (ranging from marked irritability to alarming passivity); poor eye contact; poor response to others' voices, especially to one's name being called; poor attempts at interactive play; more interest in looking at objects than people; delayed pointing to request or share; decreased to-and-fro babbling and jargoning; and lack of warm, joyful, reciprocating expressions.
>
> (p. 1195)

Early intervention is key to your child's success. Kamal Smith, a parent of a son and an autism advocate, explained,

> Seek early intervention. It is one of the most critical steps that any parent of a child with autism should take. Early intervention can help provide the learning accommodations, modifications, and services your child needs to gain autonomy, live as close to normal life as possible, and function at home and in their community.

Kamal's belief is confirmed by research. Christina Corsello (2005) reviewed early intervention programs for children with autism and summarized,

> The available evidence from a variety of programs and studies suggests that early intervention leads to better

outcomes. As we have seen, a number of studies have demonstrated that children make greater gains when they enter a program at a younger age.

(p. 82)

The National Research Council (2001) recommends children with autism receive a minimum of 25 hours of intervention per week, 12 months per year. Is your loved one with autism receiving this?

Quick Start to Support

Reflect on the question, "Where do I go from here?" In our own experiences of raising our children we recognized we parent better with a plan rather than an arbitrary approach of wandering through the years. Planning requires intentionality, and with intentionality, you move ahead with direction.

Assess where your child is *today*. How do you describe their:

Behavior? _____

Language? _____

Family relations? _____

Peer relations? _____

Learning/education? _____

Write down a quantifiable way to measure where your child is today. Next, where do you want your child to be *a year* from now? Write it down.

One year from today I want my child's:

Behavior to be _____

Language to be _____

Family relations to be _____

Peer relations to be _____

Learning/education to be _____

Now that you have a target, it is ready, set, go. Consider ABA therapy. Do you need a speech and language pathologist? What activity can your family do to create good memories? Do you need to find a social skills group or another parent with a child your child's age? Touch base with your child's teacher and get an update on their progress towards or need for an Individual Education Program (IEP). Write down and add up your child's therapy hours to determine if it's at least 25 hours per week.

Seek the Help of Professionals

You are beginning the journey of guiding your child from childhood to adulthood with the best available supports. You may need a number of services along the journey and success is about arranging the services in the right order at the right times to best position your child to learn.

For instance, you may need health care professionals if your child has feeding, digestion, or nutritional issues. If your child is not speaking or becomes frustrated when trying to communicate and resorts to problem behavior, you may need a speech and language pathologist and a behavior specialist. If making and keeping friends is a challenge, then your child may need focused social skills instruction and support. Of course, you are providing daily, on-the-spot life teachings to your child all along the way. As you create the support team to help your child, these are the most common professionals and their roles.

You will require the support of some, but not all, of the professionals listed above. Your child's unique presentation of autism will influence if or when you access these services and how you arrange your support team. Many families report the need for more professional support in the early years and less in the late teen and young adult years. Claire, a parent of an early adolescent daughter, encourages parents to "trust your instincts and urge doctors and teachers to listen and look closely at your concerns when to you share them." Shelly, a parent to a young adult son, offers this advice, "Start early, early, early and do as much therapy as you can while your child is young." Lamar describes the improvement he has seen in his teenage son by sharing, "Success occurs gradually when you have the right

TABLE 1.1 Titles and Descriptions of Common Interventionists

Professional	Role
Pediatrician	A general pediatrician oversees your child's medical care.
Developmental pediatrician	This doctor has specialized training and expertise in assessments, treatments, medical, and psychosocial development and behavior in children.
Neurologist	A neurologist has specialized training in diagnosing and treating conditions that affect the brain, nerves, and spine in children. They treat conditions including autism, cerebral palsy, epilepsy, traumatic brain injury, and more.
Behavior specialist	Commonly called behavior therapists, behavior specialists help determine when and why a child's behavior occurs and develops a plan for teaching socially acceptable replacement behaviors and related skills. Their practice is based on principles of ABA and they have specialized training and certification or are supervised by someone who does, referred to as a board certified behavior analyst (BCBA).
Occupational therapist (OT)	An occupational therapist works with children and adults to strengthen their fine motor skills, sensory motor skills, visual motor skills and to prepare them for the occupations of childhood (e.g., play) and adulthood (e.g., employment/leisure).
Physical therapist (PT)	The physical therapist helps children with motor control, posture, muscle strength, and range of motion.
Speech and language pathologist (SLP)	Commonly called speech therapists, SLPs work with children to increase their ability to express themselves through language or gestures as well as help children understand language. Speech therapy can help children correctly pronounce sounds or words and/or to use language to support social relationships. Some speech therapists also help with feeding-related issues.
Nutritionist	A nutritionist helps with your child's selective diet, helps you learn about the gut-brain connection, helps with bowel issues, and detects and advises on any nutritional deficiencies.
Special education teacher	A special education teacher has training and certification to provide direct instruction and facilitate services in the school setting that help children learn and grow in their academic, social, and independent functioning skills.

(Continued)

TABLE 1.1 (Cont.)

Professional	Role
Psychologist	The psychologist provides counseling, testing, and consultations to parents and teachers.
Psychiatrist	Psychiatrists diagnose and provide medication management and monitoring.
Respite caregiver	This person provides parents with in-home or center-based caregiving so parents have time to address their own needs and maintain healthy relationships.
Audiologist	An audiologist provides testing to determine hearing loss, function of the middle ear system, and the ability to understand speech.

treatment, with the right provider, for the right frequency per week, for the right length of time, and with hard work from you and your child."

Use your existing social supports to see where you can connect with other caregivers of children with autism. If you live close to a university, reach out to the special education department and ask if they have any groups or parent supports for autism. Bookmark the websites and resources shared throughout the chapters of this book.

Parent advocate Kamal Smith encourages other parents to document their child's journey by journaling. She explains that you don't know the future and you might end up writing a book, so document moments by writing them down. In addition, writing your feelings can be healing.

Summary

Time is valuable so start now. Give relentless pursuit to support your child and enlist the timely support of knowledgeable professionals. Use evidence-based practices that are proven to help children with autism. Connect with other parents and caregivers supporting children with autism. Trust that autism

- ◆ Is lifelong
- ◆ Affects communication, social skills, and behavior

- ◆ Occurs on a continuum from mild to severe
- ◆ Is responsive to intervention
- ◆ Has best outcomes with early and focused intervention

Raising and supporting your child with autism may not be an easy job but it is likely your most important and we will help you feel more equipped to do it. Bookmark the websites and resources shared throughout this chapter to help you help others. You've got this!

Resources

Access these quick start guide links for downloadable resources from the Florida Centers for Autism and Related Disabilities (CARD) that can be distributed to community providers to help them better understand autism and the special care and consideration that is often required in different situations.

> https://www.fau.edu/education/centersandprograms/card/documents/autismandthefaithcommunity.pdf
> http://card-usf.fmhi.usf.edu/docs/resources/CARD_ASDMH_Brochure092109.pdf
> https://www.autismontheseas.com/images/Articles/ARTICLE_-_Air_Travel_CARD.pdf
> http://card-usf.fmhi.usf.edu/docs/resources/CARD_Emergency_Room_2019_FINAL_Digital.pdf

References

American Psychiatric Association. (2013). *Diagnostic and statistical manual of mental disorders* (5th ed.). Washington, DC: American Psychiatric Association.

Corsello, C. M. (2005). Early intervention in autism. *Infants and Young Children*, *18*(2), 74–85.

Johnson, C. P., & Myers, S. M. (2007). Identification and evaluation of children with autism spectrum disorders. *Pediatrics*, *120*(5), 1183–1215.

Lord, C. (1995). Follow-up of two-year-olds referred for possible autism. *Journal of Child Psychology and Psychiatry, 36*(8), 1365–1382.

National Research Council. (2001). *Educating children with autism.* Washington, DC: National Academies Press.

2

Effective Interventions and Unproven Therapies

Effective Interventions and Unproven Therapies Explained

Navigating intervention options can be confusing and over-whelming for parents trying to act quickly but wisely to help their loved one with autism. If you don't know the best interventions to use or when to use them, you may feel stuck. Unintentionally, you might delay your child's access to essential and timely inter-ventions. Or, you may act in haste and spend your precious time and resources on interventions that are ineffective or even potentially harmful to your child. We want to help you avoid these pitfalls, by guiding you to the most up-to-date research on autism-focused interventions and highlighting a few parent-friendly interventions that can help you and your child enjoy some shared accomplishments sooner rather than later.

A Word of Caution

With the popularity of social media, celebrity blogs, and online marketing of products and services, you will encounter a lot of false information in your search for help. This information will come from sources that misleadingly call themselves "experts" and promote treatments they falsely claim to be "scientifically proven." Often, these sources will offer you a quick "recovery" or

DOI: 10.4324/9781003285953-3

a magical "cure" for autism-related challenges. As you encounter these testimonials about quick-fix treatments you may ask yourself, "what's the harm in trying?" or "what do I have to lose?" Understandably, you want to feel in control of your child's progress and will do everything in your power to make it happen.

However, it is important to remember some basic facts when making intervention decisions for your child.

♦ Autism cannot be "cured," as it is not a disease or illness
♦ Autism cannot be "out nourished," as it is not caused by only nutritional deficiencies
♦ Autism cannot be "outgrown," as it is not simply a missed milestone or two
♦ Autism cannot be "out parented," as it is not caused by poor attachment or parental neglect

Autism is neurological and lifelong. Characteristics of autism present differently from child to child and year to year, but they do not magically disappear. Decades of autism research assures us of this and we encourage you to embrace it wholeheartedly. The promotion of quick cures and fad treatments is unfair to you and unproductive for your child. It also perpetuates stigma and falsehoods that are disrespectful to the autism community as a whole. With this in mind, we urge you to proceed with caution and a healthy dose of skepticism as you navigate your way through this journey.

A Word of Encouragement

You and your child will benefit from decades of autism research and advocacy. There is better understanding of what does and does not work to address challenges that are common to individuals with autism across the life span than ever before. There is strong evidence that early and effective intervention can prevent or diminish many autism-related challenges. There are also many expert sources you can turn to again and again for guidance. So, instead of asking yourself "why not try this?" or "what are they trying?", we want you to ask, "what does the research say about addressing this specific challenge my child is having right now?" or "what is the best intervention for teaching my child this important skill now?" We will help you to answer these important questions and know when it is time to ask for help.

Understanding Evidence-Based Practices

The scientific study of autism has provided us with a list of evidence-based practices to choose from to address challenging behaviors and to teach new skills. Research has shown that the practices work again and again and can be trusted to produce positive outcomes. Put simply, there is a "menu" of options for addressing autism-specific concerns for different ages and for different purposes that is backed by years of research. Think about evidence-based practices for autism the same way you think about your child's health care.

- ◆ You decide when something can be treated by you in the home or when your child needs to be treated by a doctor
- ◆ You choose a doctor that has the certification, expertise, and experience needed to care for your child's health needs
- ◆ You will only accept medical treatments for your child that have been clinically proven safe and effective for their age
- ◆ You learn what symptoms the medicine will help and which it will not
- ◆ You are told the dose and duration of the treatment
- ◆ You are told what side effects you can expect
- ◆ You are told how long it will take before your child starts to feel better

Physicians are not the only treatment providers that need to stay up-to-date on the advances in their field to inform their practice and provide this level of detailed guidance. The same is true for the professionals who work with your child with autism. As a parent, you should know who the experts are when you need help, what you can expect from their "prescribed" interventions, and how to implement best practices in the home in their absence.

What the Research Reports

A number of professional organizations have done the hard work of sorting through what works and what does not work for you (see resources). A recent report provided by the National Clearing House for Autism Evidence Based Practices (Steinbrenner et al., 2020) summarizes 28 practices that research has demonstrated are the most effective interventions for children, youth, and adults with autism. You might consider these first-tier supports to use to help your child. In addition to describing each practice in detail, this comprehensive resource also describes the positive outcomes reported in the reviewed studies, the age groups that benefited from them, and who successfully delivered the interventions. Below is a quick reference of the categories described in this review. The full report and related resources can be found at https://autismpdc.fpg.unc.edu /how-do-i-find-out-more-about-ebps.

Unproven Therapies

When your child is sick, you make sure they take vitamins, drink a lot of fluids, eat nourishing foods, get plenty of rest, and have the comfort of the people and pets they love the most. These practices may not treat the core symptoms of your child's illness, but they do bring comfort to both you and your child in times of stress and sickness. For the core symptoms of your child's illness, you likely rely on the treatments prescribed by your pediatrician. You trust in the treatment, because you know it has been deemed safe and effective for your child's age and symptoms. You are confident that your doctor knows your child and family well and has taken your unique needs into consideration.

This is the same mindset and diligence you should have when choosing interventions to address the core social-communication and behavioral characteristics of autism. Although there are a number of second-tier interventions (dietary interventions, animal therapies) that may provide some benefit or relief for common related challenges (digestive, anxiety, sleep issues, etc.), they are not recommended in the 28 practices referenced above.

TABLE 2.1 List of Evidence-Based Practices, Outcomes, Ages and Interventionists

Evidence-based practices	Antecedent-based intervention
	Cognitive behavioral/instructional strategies
	Differential reinforcement of alternative, incompatible, or other behaviors
	Direct instruction
	Discrete trial training
	Exercise and movement
	Extinction
	Functional behavioral assessment
	Functional communication training
	Modeling
	Music-mediated intervention
	Naturalistic intervention
	Parent-implemented interventions
	Peer-mediated instruction/intervention
	Prompting
	Reinforcement
	Response interruption/redirection
	Self-management sensory integration®
	Social narratives
	Social skills training
	Task analysis
	Technology-aided instruction and intervention
	Time delay
	Video modeling
	Visual supports
Outcomes	Academic/pre-academic
	Adaptive/self-help
	Challenging/interfering behaviors
	Cognitive
	Communication
	Joint attention
	Mental health
	Motor
	Play
	Self-determination
	School readiness
	Social
	Employment
Ages	0–5 years
	6–14 years
	15–22 years
Interventionists	Behavior specialists (BCBA)
	Educators
	Parents
	Peers
	Related service providers
	Other/not specified

Many interventions also take a considerable amount of time and resources that are better spent on interventions that do work for what matters most right now to you and your child.

Examples of practices that are not evidence-based for autism-specific concerns include:

♦ Restrictive diets (e.g., gluten and casein free, dye free, etc.)
♦ Vitamin supplements
♦ Herbs and homeopathic treatments
♦ Essential oils
♦ Animal therapies (e.g., swimming with dolphins, equine therapy, etc.)
♦ Auditory integration therapy
♦ Neurofeedback therapy
♦ Rapid prompting method
♦ Chelation therapy
♦ Hyperbaric oxygen therapy
♦ Facilitated communication
♦ Attachment or holding therapies

In addition to being unsupported by research, some practices you may see on the internet or hear discussed anecdotally could be harmful to your child's health. Some are just outright dangerous. Since our goal is to steer you away from those sources, we will not list them here. Rather, we just caution you to be diligent in who you trust with your child's health and well-being. We also encourage you to always consult with trusted experts to be sure you follow the science and not the fads.

Quick Start to Using Effective Interventions

To get started quickly but smartly, you must first protect yourself and your child from misleading sources and locate trusted experts that will help you make informed intervention decisions on behalf of your child. Then, you can proceed with more confidence with interventions that are simple and safe to do on your own.

Know the Red Flags

There are some common strategies used by people marketing products and services to the autism community. These same strategies may be used to support arguments or viewpoints about autism that are not supported by science or the experts who rely on it. These include:

- ◆ Celebrity endorsements
- ◆ Pseudoscience terms like "scientifically proven," "brain-based," or "all experts agree"
- ◆ References to magical thinking, mystical claims, or vague ancient wisdom
- ◆ Terms such as "cure," "recovery," or "toxins"
- ◆ Emotional appeals (e.g., "moms who love their children…")
- ◆ Common sense appeals (e.g., "everybody knows…")
- ◆ Conspiracy theories

Dig Deeper

The same safeguards you use to ensure your child's health is treated with expert care should also be used when choosing autism interventions based on your child's unique needs. Dig deeper into the data that supports the interventions being recommended for your child. Just because something is said to work for autism, does not mean it should be assumed to work for your child. Autism is one aspect of your child. There are a number of other aspects that may impact how they respond to any given intervention. Your child's current health status, age, environments, skills, deficits, language, culture, and preferences are co-occurring conditions are all important considerations. Ask yourself and your trusted experts:

- ◆ What age does this intervention work for?
- ◆ Will it teach this specific skill, address this specific concern?
- ◆ Where is this intervention best delivered? Home? School? Clinic? All of these?
- ◆ Who should provide the intervention? Parent? Teacher? Clinician? Doctor?

◆ How much, how often, and for how long will my child likely need this intervention?
◆ What changes can I expect to see in my child? What should I look out for?
◆ How will I know if the intervention is working?
◆ My child is _____ or has _____, does this impact the effectiveness of the intervention?

Use What Works for What Matters Most

Knowing there are 28 evidence-based practices for teaching a number of skills at different ages is a good thing. However, to get started quickly you will want to start with some parent-friendly practices that you can confidently and safely use on your own. You also want to choose a few strategies to teach skills that improve daily life for you both. One recommended practice that you can start using now to increase your child's skills and independence and give you both a sense of shared accomplishment are "visual supports." A visual support is a tool that will help your child understand and navigate the social world better. Since using and understanding spoken language is challenging for children with autism, visuals are a great way to "show" instead of "tell" your child what to do.

If any of the below remind you of your child, then visual supports are a great place to start!

◆ Difficulty following daily routines
◆ Difficulty following directions
◆ Difficulty with schedule changes
◆ Difficulty transitioning between activities or settings
◆ Requires frequent redirection for attention
◆ Requires frequent reminders for behavior expectation

Visual supports are helpful and effective for:

◆ Showing daily schedules or routines
◆ Showing steps to a routine or task
◆ Showing expectations for behavior
◆ Redirecting undesired behavior

- ◆ Providing choices
- ◆ Providing alternative ways to communicate
- ◆ Providing positive reinforcement

Some good visual supports to start with are:

- ◆ Choice boards
- ◆ Token reinforcement boards
- ◆ First/then boards
- ◆ Visual schedules
- ◆ Visual checklists

Some things to keep in mind when using visual supports are:

- ◆ You will need to *model* for your child how to use the tools
- ◆ You will need to *prompt* your child to remember to use the tools
- ◆ You will need to use *reinforcement* to help your child to use them correctly and/or independently

Modeling, Prompting, and Reinforcement are *all* evidence-based practices! They are strategies that can be used in a number of ways to help your child.

- ◆ Modeling shows your child how to do something (in person or via a video demonstration)
- ◆ Prompting reminds your child of what is expected or guides them to begin or complete a task. Prompting can be verbal, visual (pointing, picture cue), or physical (guiding a hand)
- ◆ Reinforcement is your immediate response to your child's behavior or action that increases the likelihood that they will do it again

Increasing your familiarity and confidence in using these strategies correctly will go a long way. By using only these few effective practices together you can address many goals including:

- ◆ Increasing independence during daily routines (e.g., bath time, bedtime, getting dressed)
- ◆ Helping your child complete a task (e.g., putting toys away, packing school bag or lunch, setting the table, etc.)
- ◆ Decreasing anxiety or frustration about schedules or transitions (e.g., daily visual schedules, activity schedules)

To learn more about the evidence behind and step-by-step procedures for using these evidence-based practices or any of the 28 referenced here, you can access the Autism Focused Intervention Resources and Modules (AFIRM). These informative modules are free to access and are aligned with each of the practices recommended by the trusted organizations discussed here and listed in the resources.

Summary

We respect that you are your child's first and most dedicated advocate and teacher. With that in mind, we have dedicated this chapter to helping you become an informed consumer of autism-related information as well as a confident lifelong "interventionist" for your child. We hope we successfully steered you away from flashy and unfounded claims that often distract well-meaning parents. We also hope to have guided you towards the science, trusted sources, and some quick start strategies that will help you and your child start and stay on a successful path throughout your journey together.

Resources

The National Autism Center at the May Institute
https://www.nationalautismcenter.org/
The National Professional Development Center on Autism
    Spectrum Disorder
https://autismpdc.fpg.unc.edu/evidence-based-practices
The National Clearing House on Autism Evidence and Practice

https://ncaep.fpg.unc.edu/
Organization for Autism Research
https://researchautism.org/use-of-evidence-based-practices/
Autism Focused Intervention Resources and Modules (AFIRM)
https://afirm.fpg.unc.edu/afirm-modules

Reference

Steinbrenner, J. R., Hume, K., Odom, S. L., Morin, K. L., Nowell, S. W., Tomaszewski, B., … & Savage, M. N. (2020). *Evidence-based practices for children, youth, and young adults with autism.*Chapel Hill, NC: FPG Child Development Institute.

3

Medication

This is general medical information and we recommend you always work closely in conjunction with your child's health care provider. Choose a treatment that fits your child's unique needs and your family values. Most parents approach medication with caution and concern.

Medication Explained

Medication is a relatively common treatment. Mandell and colleagues (2008) found that 56% of children with autism on Medicaid took at least one medication. Nevertheless, the decision to medicate your child is often difficult and highly personal. You know your child best and, as a parent, it is hard to watch your child struggle behaviorally and socially. You are not alone when you've considered the question, "Should my child take medication?"

When reflecting on this consider these general points:

1. How is home life?
2. How is school performance?
3. How are my child's relationships?
4. Is my child hurting himself or herself?

After answering these questions, where are your thoughts? If there are concerns across multiple settings, medication might help. If there is a major concern in one area, medication might

DOI: 10.4324/9781003285953-4

help. While medication might help, maintain reasonable expectations for how it can help. South Florida developmental pediatrician Judith Aronson-Ramos, MD says,

> Medicines don't fix broken families, they don't dramatically alter IQ scores, they don't erase bad memories, and they don't instill motivation when there is none. When we understand the role medications can play, we can complement them with other interventions we need.

Since there are no medications specifically approved for autism, the best they can do is offer symptom relief. What we know about medication and autism is that:

- ◆ Medication does not cure autism
- ◆ Medication does not help every child with autism
- ◆ Currently, there are no autism specific medications
- ◆ Medication has side effects
- ◆ Medication can be expensive

What the Research Reports

Children with autism often have co-occurring disorders that complicate daily life. Dr. Emily Simonoff and colleagues (2008) studied British children with autism for co-occurring disorders. They reported that 70% of participants had at least one co-occurring disorder and 41% had two or more. Of the children in their study, the co-occurring disorders were: social anxiety (29%), attention deficit hyperactive disorder (ADHD) (28%), and oppositional defiant disorder (28%). Given the complexity of these disorders, there is no one-size-fits-all treatment and therefore a multi-modal treatment approach is needed.

Nadeau and colleagues (2011) completed a literature review to examine treatments using medication and cognitive behavioral therapy in individuals with autism and anxiety. They concluded selective serotonin-reuptake inhibitors (SSRI) medications (fluoxetine, escitalopram, fluvoxamine, paroxetine, sertraline) can help individuals with autism and anxiety, although youth with autism seemed more susceptible to adverse side effects than peers without autism. Likewise, cognitive behavioral therapy was seen to help children with autism and anxiety.

A common question for parents to ask their doctor is, "Which medication will help my child?" Lawrence Fung and colleagues (2016) systematically reviewed and analyzed the efficacy and safety of pharmacologic treatments for irritability and aggression in young people with autism. They identified forty-six randomized control trials and found Risperidone and Aripiprazole were the most effective medications. McPheeters and colleagues (2011) also conducted a review of a decade of studies on medications for children with autism. They found evidence to support

TABLE 3.1 List of Common Adverse Behaviors and Medicinal Treatments

Adverse Behavior	Possible Medicine to Treat
Hyperactive	**Stimulant medications**
Inattentive	Ritalin, Metadate, Focalin, Concerta, Daytrana,
Impulsive	Dexedrine, Vyvanse, Adderall
Difficulty focusing	**Non-stimulant medications**
	Strattera
	Intuniv
	Kapvay
	Qelbree
Depression	Zoloft
Anxiety	Paxil
Repetitive behaviors	Lexapro
Obsessive thoughts	Prozac
	Luvox
	Celexa
Irritability	Risperdal
Aggression	Abilify
Sleep problems	Geodon
Tics	Seroquel
Hyperactivity	Zyperxa
Self-injury	
Behavior problems	
Seizures	Tegretol
Moodiness	Depokate
Self-injury	Lamictal
	Topomax
	Trileptal

the benefit of Risperidone and Aripiprazole to improve behaviors in behaviors in children with autism spectrum disorder (ASD). These studies give credibility to you discussing with your child's doctor the potential benefit of using Risperidone and Aripiprazole use with your child.

The table below lists common concerning behaviors in children with ASD and the type of medication used to treat these behaviors.

Raj N. Shekhat, MD, is a board-certified child, adolescent, and adult psychiatrist at Goldcoast Psychiatry in Jupiter, Florida. His practice takes a targeted approach in working with patients and families, developing a unique treatment plan that incorporates medication and therapy. He offers a psychiatrist's perspective.

Box 3.1 Psychiatry and Autism

Psychiatry plays an integral role in the treatment of many mental health disorders. Regarding autism, in particular, psychiatry is typically part of a multi-faceted treatment plan. Including psychiatry means including psychotropic medications, which can be a difficult decision for many families. Worries about effectiveness and the risk of side effects are often the cause. Word-of-mouth and personal experience can play a key role in encouraging or dissuading parents to pursue any treatment regardless of what evidence may show.

Because each situation is unique, developing a treatment plan tailored directly to each patient and family is important. Therapy is typically a first step before medications are introduced. Specifically, Applied Behavior Analysis (ABA) therapy. ABA therapy is the gold standard for treatment, and the starting point especially in more severe forms of autism. Other more traditional forms of therapy including Cognitive Behavioral Therapy or group therapy can be included in less severe cases. Although the complexity and severity of each case is different, the inclusion of the right medication(s), therapy, and caregiver/sibling support often results in the best outcomes for patients, and their families.

Patients with autism can present additional challenges based on the diagnosis itself which may be co-occurring with any number of other mental health diagnoses, including depression, anxiety, attention deficit hyperactive disorder (ADHD), obsessive compulsive disorder (OCD), excoriation disorder (skin picking), tics, and sleep disorders. Other factors to consider are medical problems that may result in or exacerbate these psychiatric disorders. Neurological (brain), dermatological (skin), endocrine (hormonal), gynecological (hormonal), and vitamin deficiencies are among the most common co-occurring disorders that require treatment simultaneously. Often times they are missed.

The inclusion of medication is based on two main factors: severity of the illness and the impact it plays in an individual's life. A secondary factor is the impact that the symptoms and behaviors are having on family members at home. This can also help determine the severity of illness. Immediate family members can have their own lives negatively impacted with school, work, health, and relationships all being affected in varying degrees. The stress levels can often lead to other family members experiencing mental health issues themselves or an exacerbation of mental health problems they are already dealing with. Although parents and siblings should seek out support, they often go untreated.

Medications have different levels of efficacy, tolerability, dosing, and side effects. All of these factors need to be carefully weighed before making a decision of which specific medication(s) to consider and how best to proceed once a decision is made. Moreover, core features of the disorder, specifically those in regard to communication and socialization may not be directly responsive to medication.

Currently, only two medications have FDA approval in treating autism, Risperidol and Aripiprazole. Both of these medications are classified as mood stabilizers. These medications can directly improve irritability-related symptoms including aggression, tantrums, rapidly changing moods, and self-injury. Benefits must be weighed against side effects when considering any mood stabilizer medications as part of treatment. Off-label (non-FDA approved) use of medication is common in children with autism as well.

Medications in the off-label category may not have an approval for autism specifically, but can and often do have approval for co-occurring disorders in children or adults. Identifying and treating the co-occurring disorders noted earlier can have a substantial impact on the patient's mental health and ability to participate at school and at home. Oftentimes, medications are used in combination with each other, customized per individual needs, and this approach can provide better results.

Regardless of whether medications are started or not, a psychiatric assessment is a necessary first step to developing a treatment plan and knowing the full range of options available in improving the lives of those impacted by mental illness.

Quick Start to Using Medication

Unequivocally, medical professionals are the experts for prescribing. Dr. Niewiadomski-Ayala is a pediatrician and parent of a child with autism and she brings a valuable and unique perspective to her medical practice. In an interview she explained that it's often difficult to treat a five- or six-year-old with medication due to their young age. Thus, she does not immediately recommend medication and advises parents to first try approaches such as behavioral, speech, occupational, or physical therapies. If therapies don't obtain the desired results, then she considers prescribing medication, but does so with parent and teacher input. She empathizes with parents who "want their child to be like a normal child" and openly shares her expertise. She also realizes a pediatrician's limitations and if her patient is not responding well to prescribed medications, she refers to child neurologists.

Consider asking your doctor these questions:

◆ What do you recognize about my child that helps you prescribe a specific medication?
◆ What are some common side effects?
◆ Will my insurance cover the medication and if not, is there an alternative medication you can prescribe?
◆ Can this medication be rapidly stopped or is it a gradual withdrawal?
◆ If the medication comes in a pill, can it be crushed and put in applesauce or yogurt?
◆ Do you have any written information about medications?
◆ How do you monitor the medication's effectiveness?
◆ Do you have any personal experience using these medications with your own child?
◆ Would you medicate if this were your child?
◆ Can you explain to my child why he or she must take it?

Pill Swallowing

Some children with autism have difficulty swallowing pills. When this occurs, it is called pill dysphagia. Simply put, pill dysphagia is defined as "difficulty or inability to swallow pills." When this occurs, you might want to use a social narrative with your child. As described in chapter 9, a social narrative is a simple story, accompanied by pictures, that helps your child understand how to approach a new event. Below is a sample medication social narrative titled, "I Can Take My Medicine."

In conjunction with the social narrative, many parents use adaptive devices. One such device is the special cup called Oralflo for individuals four and older. According to the manufacturer's website (oralflo.com), you fill the cup half full, secure the lid, place the pill in the mouthpiece, and drink. The pill sits above the liquid on a special grill built into the lid. When the child drinks,

TABLE 3.2 Social Narrative to Assist Pill Swallowing

I can take my medicine	Image
First I open my mouth	Open mouth
Second I put the pill in my mouth	Put pill in mouth
Now I drink	Drink
Swallow fast	Swallow
I drink some more	Drink
Now I get iPad time	Use iPad

the pill and liquid enter the mouth at the same time and this prevents the pill from sticking and facilitates swallowing.

Other parents use the Pill Glide swallowing spray (flavorx.com/pill-glide/). This is available online and in retail stores. It was created by a pharmacist and to use you simply spray, place pill, drink, and swallow. Pill Glide is sugar free, dye free, gluten free, casein free, and oil free.

Medi-Straw is another tool to help individuals with pill swallowing difficulty. The Medi-Straw suspends the pill in liquid as it enters the mouth to help reduce or eliminate gagging and choking (medistraw.com).

Consider these parent provided tips to help your child take medication:

♦ First, place liquid in mouth, slightly tilt your child's head back, drop in the pill. They swallow
♦ Put the pill inside a gusher
♦ Get a can of spray whip cream. Place pill on tongue, give squirt of whip cream which keeps pill in place. Your child swallows

- ◆ Chew some food, like a cracker or piece of bread, and then place the capsule on the tongue just as your child is about to swallow the food
- ◆ Give the medication first thing in the morning when he is super thirsty and the pill goes right down
- ◆ Provide lots of rewards much like when potty training
- ◆ Demonstrate swallowing a small bean and not tic tacs, because candy often has a good taste

Summary

While medication can help your child, it is only one part of your child's treatment plan. Work with your medical professional to determine the best medication and schedule for your child and continue to teach your child the skills that pills can't teach.

Resources

Autism Intervention Research Network on Physical Health
https://airpnetwork.ucla.edu/
American Academy of Child and Adolescent Psychiatry: Autism Spectrum Disorder Parents' Medication Guide
https://www.aacap.org/App_Themes/AACAP/Docs/resource _centers/autism/Autism_Spectrum_Disorder_Parents_ Medication_Guide.pdf
National Institute of Child Health and Human Development: Medication Treatment for Autism
https://www.nichd.nih.gov/health/topics/autism/condition-info/treatments/medication-treatment

References

Fung, L. K., Mahajan, R., Nozzolillo, A., Bernal, P., Krasner, A., Jo, B., ... & Hardan, A. Y. (2016). Pharmacologic treatment of severe irritability and problem behaviors in autism: a systematic review and meta-analysis. *Pediatrics*, *137*(Supplement_2), S124–S135.

Mandell, D. S., Morales, K. H., Marcus, S. C., Stahmer, A. C., Doshi, J., & Polsky, D. E. (2008). Psychotropic medication use among Medicaid-enrolled children with autism spectrum disorders. *Pediatrics*, *121*(3), e441–e448. https://doi.org/10.1542/peds.2007-0984.

McPheeters, M. L., Warren, Z., Sathe, N., Bruzek, J. L., Krishnaswami, S., Jerome, R. N., & Veenstra-VanderWeele, J. (2011). A systematic review of medical treatments for children with autism spectrum disorders. *Pediatrics*, *127*(5), e1312–e1321.

Nadeau, J., Sulkowski, M. L., Ung, D., Wood, J. J., Lewin, A. B., Murphy, T. K., … Storch, E. A. (2011). Treatment of comorbid anxiety and autism spectrum disorders. *Neuropsychiatry*, *1*(6), 567–578. https://doi.org/10.2217/npy.11.62.

Simonoff, E., Pickles, A., Charman, T., Chandler, S., Loucas, T., & Baird, G. (2008). Psychiatric disorders in children with autism spectrum disorders: Prevalence, comorbidity, and associated factors in a population-derived sample. *Journal of the American Academy of Child and Adolescent Psychiatry*, *47*(8), 921–929. https://doi.org/10.1097/CHI.0b013e318179964f.

4

Supplements and Nutrition

Supplements and Nutrition Explained

You've heard the saying, "What you eat matters," so undoubt-edly you understand your child's nutrition is important. Adults and children need the same type of nutritional intake of vitamins and minerals as good nutrition leads to good health. But when it comes to autism, you've likely asked yourself, "What type of nutrition is best for my child?" Your child might be an extremely picky eater with a limited range of foods. His selectivity might require you to create a special meal just for him while the family eats the nightly meal. A limited food intake can result in your child not obtaining all nutrients necessary for healthy growth as well as creating unwanted health problems.

Healthy nutrition also contributes to maintaining a healthy gastrointestinal (GI) system so kids with poor nutrition often have gastrointestinal sensitivities. Some children with chronic feeding problems are at risk for slower growth, developmental delays, psychological deficits, and poor academic achievement. A healthy GI system often equates to healthy living.

While you don't have to become a licensed professional, understanding nutrition positions you to help your child. We offer general nutrition advice and recommend you consult with your medical professional or a registered nutritionist as the ben-efits of nutrition as a "treatment" for autism are largely ineffec-tive and somewhat controversial. Nutrition and supplements

DOI: 10.4324/9781003285953-5

alone have not been proven in large scale research to improve the core symptoms of autism: social deficits, communication deficits, restricted interest, and repetitive behaviors. However, our position is that adequate and well-balanced nutritional intake is an underlying component for helping some of the co-occurring issues your child might have such as gastrointestinal problems.

What the Research Reports

Overall, large scale independent research has not established that nutrition is an effective evidence-based practice, as you might recall it was not included in the Evidence-Based Practice for Children, Youth, and Young Adults with Autism report as one of the 28 best practices referenced in Chapter 2. Yet, nutrition is important when taking a whole-child perspective for helping one obtain a positive quality of life. The takeaway from the meta-analysis studies discussed below suggests that you should "proceed with caution," as you don't want to exclude doing what is most effective using evidence-based practices in the hope that a nutritional change was the missing link.

Eating is an essential life-activity, and when we eat, we must excrete. Gastrointestinal disorders rank among the most common medical conditions associated with autism. In a 2014 meta-analysis, Barbara McElhanon and colleagues (2014) reported children with autism experienced more GI symptoms, higher rates of diarrhea, constipation, and abdominal pain. It's often the child's selective diet that produces some of these symptoms. And, if you have personally had an upset stomach, constipation, or GI issues, you will understand just how much they affect your concentration and behavior. You can thwart some of these problems with adequate nutrition.

Patricia Esteban-Figueroa and colleagues (2019) completed a meta-analysis examining the food consumption and nutritional intake of children with autism and typically developing children. They concluded, "Children with ASD in this meta-analysis showed a significantly lower intake of protein, calcium, phosphorus, selenium, vitamin D, thiamine, riboflavin, and vitamin B12 and a significantly higher intake of polyunsaturated fatty acids and vitamin E in comparison to typically developing children" (p. 1093). In addition, the children with ASD had lower consumption of omega-3 fatty acids and ate higher levels of fruits and vegetables than typically developing children. However, the authors included a caution about these findings given relatively few studies were found to include in their analyses.

Spark and colleagues' meta-analysis confirmed that children with autism have more feeding problems compared with peers. They reported a lower intake of calcium and protein and higher levels of nutritional inadequacies in children with ASD.

A meta-analysis by Fraguas and colleagues indicated dietary supplements showed global improvement in children with autism but did not reveal a recommendation of a specific dietary intervention. Of the supplements reviewed, the use of omega-3 supplementation was more successful than placebos for improving symptoms related to anxiety, behavior, impulsivity, stereotypes, and restricted and repetitive behaviors, but the effect size was small, which makes the likelihood of this helping your child quite limited.

Kanwaljit Singh and colleagues (2014) conducted an interesting study using phytochemical sulforaphane, which is derived from broccoli sprout extracts. They compared its effectiveness to a placebo in children with ASD. There was daily oral dosing for 18 weeks followed by 4 weeks without treatment. They evaluated effectiveness using rating scales. At the end of the study, Singh reported a 17–34% improvement in subjects' behavior whereas the placebo group had minimal improvements.

Special diets for autism are controversial and not supported by large scale research. Karhu and colleagues (2020) studied nutritional interventions for ASD including a gluten-free and casein-free diet, a ketogenic diet, probiotics, a specific carbohydrate diet, polyunsaturated fatty acids supplements, vitamin A, C, B12, B6, and magnesium supplements, as well as folic acid supplements. They recognized that there was no conclusive evidence for a standard treatment nutritional therapy and concluded, "Despite these methodological drawbacks, studies indicate that nutritional interventions can be used as an adjuvant treatment to usual first-line therapies, which include speech and language therapy, occupational therapy, applied behavioral therapy, and educational programs" (p. 14).

Vitamin B6 and magnesium, vitamin B12, vitamin D3, omega-3 fatty acids, and Folinic acid were examined by Li and colleagues (2018). They reviewed studies containing these five supplements for nutritional deficits in children with ASD. Of the five supplements, Vitamin B6 and magnesium were not recommended. The authors found inconclusive but acceptable support for B12, vitamin D3, and omega 3s. Folinic acid was a promising recommendation. Like most studies, further research was recommended since there was no conclusive evidence that these supplements would reduce the core autism symptoms in your child.

In summary, these meta-analyses studies suggest that nutrition and supplements alone are not a sufficient treatment but might provide improvement for some individuals. The supplements used were varied and one supplemental approach could not be recommended for all. Based on these meta-analyses, the use of nutritional products appears to carry minimal risks and does not have enough evidence to support improvement in the core symptoms of autism.

Quick Start to Using Supplements and Nutrition

Let's start with the generally recommended guidelines and nutrition basics. The 2020–2025 dietary guidelines for Americans are found at dietaryguidelines.gov. For children aged two and older, the recommended guidelines for consumption include:

- ◆ Vegetables of all types—dark green; red and orange; beans, peas, and lentils; starch; and other vegetables
- ◆ Fruits, especially whole fruit
- ◆ Grains, at least half of which are whole grain
- ◆ Dairy, including fat-free or low-fat milk, yogurt, and cheese, and/or lactose-free versions and fortified soy beverages and yogurt as alternatives

♦ Protein foods, including lean meats, poultry, and eggs; seafood; beans, peas, and lentils; and nuts, seeds, and soy products
♦ Oils, including vegetable oils and oils in food, such as seafood and nuts

We know that healthy eating helps maintain our healthy body weight and reduces the risk of developing health conditions including type 2 diabetes, iron deficiency, and cavities. The caveat is that our kids with autism do not share this well-rounded viewpoint on the benefit of eating a balanced diet! They often have a strong opinion about eating what they like and liking what they eat. Our kids often have issues with:

♦ Sensory textures of foods
♦ Flavors, tastes, colors, and smells of foods
♦ Chewing or swallowing difficulties
♦ Unpleasant power struggles during mealtime
♦ Previously associating certain foods with stomach pain and discomfort

Kids with autism often have food neophobia, which is the fear of new foods. This is different from being a picky eater, as picky eaters are generally reluctant to eat specific foods. A child's food neophobia leads to behaviors which might include shutting down, avoidance, self-stimulating, or tantrums. This causes many parents to keep the peace and stick with an imbalanced diet of serving what your child eats and supplementing when you can.

Nutritional concerns often lead parents to approach the pediatrician for advice. When you discuss nutrition with your pediatrician, your child's doctor might begin with basics including:

♦ Discussing history
♦ Discussing behavioral interventions
♦ A physical exam
♦ Ordering a laboratory evaluation of blood, urine, and stool

This approach helps determine a metabolic profile, vitamin levels, peptides, toxins, and pathogens. Your pediatrician will review the results to determine proteins, deficiencies, and infections. Depending on the results, you might ask, "What's next?" Your pediatrician might refer you to a pediatric gastroenterologist, ear, nose, and throat specialist, or a speech and language therapist specializing in swallowing difficulties.

Some families choose to work with an integrative medicine doctor who examines underlying multi-factorial causes of conditions that commonly occur with autism. These types of doctors complete the above as well as include:

◆ Discussing probiotics
◆ Digestive enzymes
◆ Identification and removal of problem foods
◆ Suggestions for replacing the problem foods with equivalent nutrients
◆ Meal suggestions
◆ Supplements
◆ Behavior therapy to expand your child's food intake

A few internet resources for locating nutritional professionals and resources include:

◆ nutritionistnear.me
◆ healthprofs.com/us/nutritionists-dietitians/autism
◆ eatright.org for registered dietician nutritionists

We recommend you avoid working with any doctor that promotes 'curing' autism.

James Adams, PhD, is currently a President's Professor at Arizona State University, where he heads the Autism/Asperger's Research Program to conduct autism research. He is also on the board for the Autism and Nutritional Research Center and published a Top 10 Nutritional Recommendations for ASD. This list provides a quick start way to embark on your nutritional journey. The Autism and Nutritional Research Center recommends you tend to these 10 items.

Box 4.1 Top Ten Recommendations for Nutritional Supplementation for Children and Adults with Autism/Asperger's

By James B. Adams, PhD
Director, Autism/Asperger's Research Program
Arizona State University

1) **Healthy diet:**
   3–4 servings of healthy vegetables (especially leafy greens)
   1–2 servings of fruit (especially whole fruit)
   1–2 servings of protein
   Minimal sugar, junk food
   Avoid artificial colors, flavors, preservatives
2) **Trial of gluten-free, casein-free diet**—1 month for casein, 3 months for gluten
3) **Vitamin/mineral supplement**—ANRC Essentials or similar brand
4) **Check iron and vitamin D status:**

   Iron: Low iron is especially common in individuals with sleep problems, young children, and females who are menstruating. Add iron if needed—but only if needed, as too much iron can also be a problem
   Vitamin D: A blood test can detect if a person has low vitamin D—this is common if people have less than 1 hour per day of direct exposure to the sun. Windows, clothing, and sunscreen lotion block most of the sunlight needed to make vitamin D

5) **Essential fatty acids**—especially needed if not eating 1 serving of fatty fish each week
6) **Amino acids**—especially if consuming insufficient protein
7) **Carnitine**—especially if not eating 2 or more servings/week of beef or pork
8) **Digestive enzymes**—especially if loose stools or gaseousness
9) **Melatonin**—if having problems sleeping
10) **Trial of very high dose vitamin B6 with Mg**—8 mg B6 per 10 pounds bodyweight, and half that for magnesium; i.e., for a 100-pound person, 800 mg B6 and 400 mg magnesium

For more information on the treatments listed above, see Summary of Dietary, Nutritional, and Medical Treatments for Autism—based on over 150 published research articles—by James B. Adams, PhD, http://autism.asu.edu.

Dr. Adams' team provided guidance for a research-based, 120-day Autism Nutritional Research Center protocol to provide a child with comprehensive nutritional support. To supervise you in this process, their website (autismnrc.org) provides contact information for physicians and nutritionists familiar with special diets and nutritional supplements for children with autism.

Dr. Judith Aronson-Ramos is a developmental pediatrician in south Florida and she supports parents of children with autism. She understands autism from the professional and parent perspective and is a realist about using diet as a "treatment" for autism. She provided a concise summary of her principles of healthy eating for children with autism.

Box 4.2 Special Diets for ASD

By Judith Aronson-Ramos, MD

You are what you eat was a popular expression in the 1970s. Throughout the centuries, foods have been used as medicine. No doubt, diet and the quality of what people consume matter in health and longevity. However, do we have the knowledge at this point in time to say with certainty that a diet can "cure" autism? At the present time, there isn't a single specialized diet proven to treat autism spectrum disorders. There is information on the internet, in books, workshops, and promoted by physicians, researchers, and parents that in certain populations of children with autism spectrum disorders, dietary changes do make a big difference in their children's lives. There is plenty of good reason to debate and scrutinize the pros and cons of these claims. What we can say with some certainty at this point is that diets do matter for *some children* with autism, and diets do matter for the optimal functioning of all human beings. **However, the extent to which dietary changes can make a difference in the lives of children with autism should not be overstated.**

Many of us in the field of treating children and adolescents in the autism spectrum know there is not one type of autism, but *many autisms*. Given this reality, where one child may respond to a dietary manipulation, another may not. This is what parents will tell you as well. A casein and gluten free diet, soy free and yeast free diet, or elimination diets of different kinds may have resulted in significant improvement for one family and imperceptible change for another. What the research shows at this point is that children with significant gastrointestinal problems—constipation, diarrhea, abdominal pain, irregularity—these children seem to benefit the most from dietary interventions. However, there is no specific dietary intervention, including casein and gluten free, which has rigorous science to back it up. There may be some research but it is generally not of sufficient quality to validate use of the diet by most medical professionals. Parents that want to trial different diets can and do, which is certainly their choice. However, my advice is to be sure your child has properly balanced nutrition—fats, carbohydrates, and proteins of good quality. Also, be sure your child is not experiencing any psychological distress from feeling deprived of favorite foods. Many families want to do *something* to improve nutrition and hedge their bets on using dietary interventions which may at least positively contribute to improving the symptoms of their child with ASD, and **this should be honored and respected when it is done wisely and safely.**

What we do know at this point is that some children are sensitive to specific foods, dyes, and preservatives. It also only makes sense that eating poorly—a lot of junk food, refined carbohydrates, and excessively processed foods— is not conducive to good physical or neurological health. What I recommend are certain practices of healthy eating which are not restrictive and may benefit the ASD child or adolescent. This includes the following principles:

1. Eat clean whole foods—this means shopping the periphery of the grocery store more than the aisles. Eat fruits, vegetables, nuts, seeds, meat, fish, cheese, yogurt, and essentially real foods.
2. Avoid preservatives, dyes, trans-fats, high fructose corn syrup, and additives where possible. If you can eat organic this may be preferable, though this has not been of proven benefit either. However, eating organic often eliminates many of the ingredients in processed foods you want to avoid, so it does simplify shopping.
3. Include the "super foods" in your diet. These foods have well documented health benefits as anti-oxidants, improved immune function, enhanced neurological functioning, lowering cholesterol, and more. You can

be creative in how these foods are served and prepared to get your children to eat them ... good for parents, too! There is bound to be something on this list for everyone:

- Beans, Blueberries, Broccoli, Oats, Oranges, Pumpkin, Salmon, Soy, Spinach, Tea (green or black), Tomatoes, Turkey, Walnuts, Yogurt

4. Be sure your child is ingesting enough protein in the day, this means with breakfast and lunch. Many children are protein free throughout their day, eating mostly carbohydrates—bagels, waffles, and cereal for breakfast; pasta, pizza, and salad for lunch. These are low protein meals. Encourage at least a small amount of protein—equivalent to the size of your child's fist— with all meals, especially breakfast and lunch. This means at breakfast including foods such as eggs, yogurt, nuts, high protein cereals and breads, energy bars with protein, smoothies with protein powder, and healthy breakfast meats (turkey, sausage, and bacon, etc.). Lunch ideally should have a protein source—a turkey sandwich, even PBJ on whole grain bread, healthy lunch meats, tuna—sparingly, high protein pasta, bean burrito, etc. It can be done! School-bought lunches are bound to be a bust, unless you have a cafeteria offering healthy choices.

5. Avoid sugary and caffeinated drinks. These cause high peaks and troughs in insulin production and will impair concentration and focus.

6. Use healthy fats—these are non-hydrogenated unsaturated or polyunsaturated fats, which don't clog arteries and lead to improved cerebrovascular (brain blood flow), as well as cardiovascular effects. Good fats: olive oil, canola oil, peanut oil, and corn oil. Bad fats: butter, coconut oil, and palm oil. Research does show that

certain fats, such as omega-3 fatty acids, reduce inflammation and may help lower the risk of certain chronic diseases. Omega-3 fatty acids are highly concentrated in the brain and are important for cognitive performance and behavioral function. Taking an omega-3 fatty acid supplement may be beneficial.

7. Anti-oxidants in plentiful quantities in the form of fruits, vegetables, and beans. Here is the list of the top foods with the most anti-oxidant power: pinto and red beans, blueberries, cranberries, raspberries, strawberries, apples, pecans, plums, russet potatoes, and artichoke hearts. You will notice there is a lot of overlap with the super foods. Remember an anti-oxidant plays the role in the body of defending against inflammation and oxidative stress, which can damage DNA and various cellular processes. Because we do not entirely know the mechanism of how and why ASD occurs, and there is the potential that immune mechanisms and problems with detoxification at the cellular level may play a role, it is reasonable to eat a diet rich in anti-oxidants.

8. Dietary enzyme supplements are popular with some families and their benefit has yet to be determined. I do not recommend them on a routine basis.

9. Dietary supplements are fraught with controversy, and loaded with extensive claims.

The special diets and supplements can quickly become a plethora of confusing information. It's refreshing that a key takeaway point from Drs. Adams and Aronson-Ramos is for your child to eat healthy vegetables and protein. You can handle that! We address how to help your child eat more foods in Chapter 10 on Toilet Training, Feeding, and Sleeping.

Summary

It's promising to know that you have control over your child's nutrition. Start with the basics of nutrition and then examine the above principles as they relate to your child. If your child has unknown food intolerances, it is worth doing a deep dive to understand nutrition. While supplements and diets aren't treatments for autism, some hold promise for individual improvement of co-occurring conditions. However, it is important to consider your child's health and eating habits when deciding to remove foods from an already limited diet, or add foods that might complicate any existing digestive-related challenges. We've outlined some steps you can take on your own as well as some follow-up resources. Some parents choose an independent path while others work with nutritionists or doctors. What is your next step?

Resources

American Heart Association
https://www.heart.org/en/healthy-living/healthy-eating/
    eat-smart/nutrition-basics/dietary-recommendations-for
    -healthy-children
Healthy Children.org
https://www.healthychildren.org/English/Pages/default.aspx
National Institute of Child Health and Human Development:
    Nutritional Therapy for Autism
https://www.nichd.nih.gov/health/topics/autism/condition-
    info/treatments/nutritional-therapy

References

Esteban-Figuerola, P., Canals, J., Fernández-Cao, J. C., & Arija Val, V. (2019). Differences in food consumption and nutritional intake between children with autism spectrum disorders and typically developing children: A meta-analysis. *Autism, 23*(5), 1079–1095. https://doi.org /10.1177/1362361318794179.

Karhu, E., Zukerman, R., Eshraghi, R. S., Mittal, J., Deth, R. C., Castejon, A. M., ... & Eshraghi, A. A. (2020). Nutritional interventions for autism spectrum disorder. *Nutrition Reviews*, *78*(7), 515–531. https://doi.org/10.1093/nutrit/nuz092.

Li, Y. J., Li, Y. M., & Xiang, D. X. (2018). Supplement intervention associated with nutritional deficiencies in autism spectrum disorders: A systematic review. *European Journal of Nutrition*, *57*(7), 2571–2582. https://doi.org/10.1007/s00394-017-1528-6.

McElhanon, B. O., McCracken, C., Karpen, S., & Sharp, W. G. (2014). Gastrointestinal symptoms in autism spectrum disorder: A meta-analysis. *Pediatrics*, *133*(5), 872–883. https://doi.org/10.1542/peds.2013-3995.

Singh, K., Connors, S. L., Macklin, E. A., Smith, K. D., Fahey, J. W., Talalay, P., & Zimmerman, A. W. (2014). Sulforaphane treatment of autism spectrum disorder (ASD). *Proceedings of the National Academy of Sciences*, *111*(43). https://doi.org/10.1073/pnas.1416940111.

5

Applied Behavior Analysis

Applied Behavior Analysis (ABA) Explained

ABA is commonly referred to as "behavior therapy." However, ABA is more than a therapeutic approach. It is a science we have learned to use in applied settings for the purpose of addressing behaviors that are socially significant for children, adolescents, and adults. We will help you understand how this science works, so you and your child can benefit from it.

Understanding Problem Behavior

Many children with autism display a number of problem behaviors when they are frustrated or upset. Despite parents' best efforts, children with autism are not easily redirected or consoled in these moments and they can remain upset for long periods of time after. However, it is important to note that autism, in itself, does not cause problem behavior. Nor are parents of children with autism somehow less equipped to manage challenging behaviors that are common in young children.

Not all children with autism will have behaviors that a parent will deem unmanageable or warrant professional help. However, when a child has difficulty expressing their needs effectively or is unable to manage their own discomfort or frustration, problem behaviors are likely to arise. At these times, you may feel like there is little choice but to respond to problem behavior by granting their child's requests or protests in the moment they occur. It

DOI: 10.4324/9781003285953-6

is often the only way to meet their needs, relieve their distress, and keep them safe. It is common for this pattern of responding to begin in early childhood when many of these behaviors are considered "developmentally appropriate."

However, for children with autism, problem behaviors often become more frequent and intense over time and can carry over to new environments (school, play groups) and people (teachers, peers). This can be both frustrating and frightening. Therefore, you may try to avoid any environment and/or people that are likely to trigger your child's problem behavior. In turn, your child may miss out on opportunities to adapt to new people and places. You may also begin to feel more and more isolated. For these reasons, children with autism often require more focused intervention than parents are accustomed to providing on their own.

Understanding ABA

ABA is recognized as the "gold standard" approach for children with autism (Foxx, 2008). So, you may have received a professional or "word-of-mouth" referral for ABA services when your child was first diagnosed or know families who use ABA services. However, as much as there is an increased awareness of behavior therapeutic services within the autism community, less is understood about how ABA differs from less systematic approaches, as well as what constitutes high quality ABA services. So, let us begin by addressing some common questions posed by parents when deciding if ABA services are a good fit for their family.

- ◆ **"Is ABA only for young children with ASD?"** No, ABA does not treat only one population or age group. Although it is highly effective for children with autism and early intervention is best, adolescents and adults with and without disabilities have greatly benefited from ABA services

- ◆ **"Does ABA only treat problem behavior?"** No, ABA is effective at reducing problem behavior and this is often a priority for treatment. However, ABA also teaches a number of socially significant skills. Some common areas addressed include:

◆ Self-regulation skills: calming strategies, tolerating/communicating discomfort
◆ Social skills: greetings, responding to social interactions, play skills, turn-taking
◆ Safety skills: preventing elopement, buckling car seat/seatbelt, pedestrian skills
◆ Daily living skills: feeding, sleeping, bathing, toileting, completing routines
◆ Academic skills: writing, reading, counting
◆ **"Is ABA too cold/robotic for children?"** No, it is true that ABA is a structured and systematic approach. However, ABA programs are designed to be highly engaging/motivating for children. Much of ABA service provision is play-based and child-led
◆ **"Does ABA bribe children into behaving better?"** No, the power of reinforcement is a core principle of ABA. However, reinforcement should not be confused with bribery. Bribery takes place before a child engages in an appropriate behavior or after the child engages in inappropriate behavior. Reinforcement occurs only after the child has engaged in an appropriate behavior and is done so with careful planning and intention
◆ **"Is ABA just hours of table work?"** No, ABA is not a "one size fits all" approach. ABA uses a combination of instructional methods tailored to the learner's specific needs, preferences, and environment. Some common approaches include:
◆ Discrete trial training: 1:1 method that breaks down complex skills into discrete steps and provides repeated opportunities for instruction, modeling, practice, feedback, and reinforcement
◆ Incidental teaching: Learning opportunities are structured into the child's natural environment using the child's own interests and motivations to lead the intervention
◆ Pivotal response training: Child-led/play-based intervention that focuses on the development of "pivotal" skill

domains including motivation, initiating social interactions, self-regulation, and responding to multiple cues
◆ Functional communication training: Replaces problem behavior (aggression, etc.) or subtle behavior (hand leading, etc.) with a more appropriate form of communication (verbal or nonverbal)
◆ **"Where are ABA services provided?"** Professional ABA services are delivered in clinics, homes, schools, and in the community. Since children with ASD often have difficulty generalizing skills to new places and people, skills are taught and/or practiced in the environment in which they are expected to occur whenever possible
◆ **"Who provides professional ABA services?"** ABA is practiced under the supervision of a board certified behavior analyst (BCBA), the required credential specific to this field. Although services may be implemented regularly by a registered behavioral therapist (RBT), the BCBA maintains an ongoing presence throughout treatment. The BCBA is responsible for:
◆ Selecting target behaviors to decrease and/or increase
◆ Observing behavior to determine when and why it occurs
◆ Overseeing the development and implementation of a behavior intervention plan
◆ Developing a data collection plan to monitor progress
◆ Analyzing data to determine if any modifications to the plan are needed
◆ Communicating progress and addressing any questions/concerns
◆ **What role should I expect to play in my child's ABA services?"** Parent training is key to the success of any well-developed ABA program. Children benefit most from ABA services when parents participate to the greatest extent possible. Effective behavior intervention strategies should be explained and modeled for parents. Opportunities to practice and receive feedback should be provided to parents, so they can confidently and effectively use the same strategies in the absence of their service providers

What the Research Reports

Over the past 40 years, a large body of research has shown the effectiveness of ABA procedures to reduce problem behavior and teach skills to individuals with autism across their lifespan (National Clearinghouse on Autism Evidence and Practice [NCAEP]). ABA works because it is both a science and a practice. That is, the methods used in the provision of ABA services (the practice) are based on scientific principles of behavior that govern how we *all* learn to interact with each other and our environment over time (the science) (Baer, Wolf, & Risley, 1968). To be active participants in ABA services, it is important for parents to understand the basic scientific principles upon which the practices are based. The following provides a summary of the science that informs behavior intervention.

ABCs of Behavior

A foundational principle of ABA is the understanding that behavior is shaped by the environment. To understand when and why problem behavior happens, we must observe not only your child, but also the events that occur before and after the behavior of concern. This systematic observation of behavior in your child's natural environment is referred to as "ABC analysis" (Antecedent-Behavior-Consequence). Using ABC analysis, we look for the following patterns in the child's behavior:

◆ **Antecedent**: An antecedent is anything that occurs in the environment immediately before a behavior. By observing antecedents, we can identify what "triggers" the behavior in a given setting. Once you can identify what triggers your child's behavior, you can better predict when and where it is likely to occur. Only then, can you learn to introduce effective preventative strategies (Antecedent Interventions)

◆ **Behavior**: To successfully change behavior, we need to first define it in objective, observable and measurable terms. By doing so, we avoid judgmental terms such as "acting out," which suggests your child is making an active choice to misbehave. We also avoid vague terms such as "non-compliance" or "tantrum," which can vary greatly from child to child. This is known as an "operational definition." For example, rather than defining behavior as a "tantrum," an operational definition might be "any instance in which your child throws herself to the ground in tears." This more aptly describes what your child's specific behavior looks and sounds like and discriminates it from similar looking/sounding behaviors (falling to floor/squealing with laughter). This allows for a more accurate measurement of the behavior before and after intervention. Without this operational definition, it would be difficult to determine what specific behavior is being addressed by the intervention team and whether or not their efforts are having the desired effect on the behavior over time (reduced or increased frequency/ duration)

◆ **Consequence**: A consequence is any change that occurs in the environment immediately following a behavior. From an ABA perspective, a consequence is not synonymous with something negative. Rather, consequences are observed in a neutral way. A consequence can be either intentional or unintentional. In ABC analysis, we are not concerned with the "intention" of actions, only the "effect" actions have on future behavior. Consequences are observed to determine two important variables that impact future behavior:

◆ Whether something is added (**positive**) or removed (**negative**) from the environment as a result of the behavior

◆ Whether the behavior is more likely to occur again in the future based on something being added or removed (**reinforcement**) or if it is less likely to occur again in the future based on something being added or removed (**punishment**)

It is important to note that what reinforces behavior (increases) or punishes behavior (decreases) cannot be assumed, only observed. What is reinforcing for one child can be punishing for another. What reinforces one behavior, could punish another. Consider a common experience amongst parents, the grocery store meltdown. The child is told they will have to leave a toy they excitedly pulled off the shelf behind (antecedent). Immediately after, the child throws themselves to the ground in tears (the behavior). The parent wants to quiet the child quickly, so she puts the toy into the grocery basket (consequence). Again, the parent tries to remove the toy prior to checkout (antecedent). The child flops to the ground in tears, louder this time (behavior). The parent sighs and gives the child the toy to avoid embarrassment (consequence).

Although the parent's intention was to stop the problem behavior not encourage it, she inadvertently provided "positive reinforcement" for the behavior in both instances by providing the child access to the toy each time. By observing behavior-consequence sequences in this way, you can learn the purpose of your child's behavior. Only then, can you make effective changes to how you will respond to problem behavior in the future (Consequence Interventions) and, more importantly, learn what you can teach your child to do instead.

Functional Behavior Assessment (FBA)

Another foundational principle of ABA is the understanding that all behavior serves a function. In simplest terms, there is a purpose for why we behave how we do when we do. Rather than choosing between "good" and "bad" behavior, we behave in ways that get our needs and wants met efficiently and consistently. All behavior can be interpreted as serving four main functions:

◆ **Sensory/automatic reinforcement:** Sensory seeking or avoiding actions
◆ **Escape/avoidance:** Delay or eliminate something unwanted/aversive
◆ **Attention:** Access social engagement or access something that is socially mediated
◆ **Tangible:** Access a preferred item/activity

A single behavior can serve multiple functions. For example, your child may hit a sibling to gain access to a toy (tangible) or they might hit you when required to initiate a bedtime routine (escape/avoidance). The function of a behavior can also change over time. Initially, a child might scream to block out a loud or aversive noise (sensory/automatic reinforcement). As screaming is likely to result in a quick response from a caregiver, screaming may subsequently serve the function of gaining attention quickly.

The formal process for determining the most likely function(s) of a given behavior, is called a Functional Behavior Assessment (FBA). An FBA is comprised of a series of structured interviews with people most familiar with the child and direct observation of the child's behavior in context with the environment in which it occurs (ABC analysis).

Behavior Intervention Plans (BIP)

As important as it is to understand why problem behavior occurs through the FBA process, it is equally important to identify a plan for teaching a more appropriate but "functionally equivalent" behavior your child can do in its place. In ABA, this is referred to as a "replacement behavior." Without a replacement behavior, problem behavior will inevitably persist. In the beginning, replacement behaviors must:

- ◆ Serve the same function as the problem behavior (sensory, escape, attention, tangible?)
- ◆ Be systematically taught (incidental teaching, functional communication training?)
- ◆ Be frequently modeled for the child (what does it look like when done correctly?)
- ◆ Be prompted (what verbal/nonverbal cue will they need in the moment?)
- ◆ Be reinforced quickly and consistently (how will they know it works as well?)

When a functionally equivalent replacement behavior is identified, then a behavior intervention plan can be developed and implemented. The BIP should specifically describe:

◆ The function(s) of the target behavior(s)
◆ Operational definitions for the target and replacement behavior(s)
◆ Strategies/procedures that will be used to prevent problem behavior (antecedent strategies)
◆ Instructional methods for teaching the replacement behavior(s)
◆ How reinforcement will be delivered consistently for replacement behaviors and prevented consistently for problem behaviors (consequence strategies)
◆ How progress will be monitored and reported

When you work with a Board Certified Behavior Analyst, they take the lead in understanding your concerns and your child's needs to do a formal Functional Behavior Assessment and create the Behavior Intervention Plan. However, you can apply these principles too.

Quick Starts to Using Applied Behavior Analysis

Some behaviors warrant immediate intervention by professionals with specialized expertise (see "When to Get Help"). For others, you can begin to embed ABA principles and practices into your existing family routines to improve the quality of day-to-day life for you and your child. Below are some feasible first steps you can take to think and react differently to problem behavior when it arises.

Think Like a Scientist

Yes, this is easier said by professionals than done by parents. It is understood that you are emotionally invested in how your child is perceived and received by others. It is also understood that you are tired/frustrated by problem behavior that persists despite your best efforts. However, thinking about the scientific principles that drive behavior, is an important first step to facilitating sustainable behavior change. Think about your child's problem behavior as a form of communication. Problem behavior communicates a skill deficit (something your child cannot do), a motivational deficit (something your child does not want to do), or a combination of both. Often, problem behavior is exhausting and requires a lot of effort on the part of your child. If they could do something else to achieve the same results consistently with less effort – they likely would choose to do so. Before engaging with your child's problem behavior, take a step back and ask yourself, "what is this behavior communicating to me" and more importantly "how can my child communicate it more appropriately?"

Remember your ABCs

You may have the desire to address all behaviors at once. Or, you may feel overwhelmed and not know where to begin. Take a deep breath and let yourself off the hook for tackling all things at once. It is best to prioritize one behavior, one time of day, or even one routine to begin.

First, take an honest inventory of your child's behaviors and the routines that are most impacted by behavior challenges. Consider how you might complete the following statement: "If only _____ occurred less, then _____ would be so much easier/more enjoyable." Choose a behavior that is safe to address on your own and one you are comfortable addressing at this point in time. Take a moment to define your chosen behavior in observable and measurable terms. This will help you stay focused only on the behavior of concern in the moment and help you discriminate it from others. You will also be more cognizant of how the behavior might change over time.

Next, conduct your own "ABC" analysis to better understand when and why the behavior of focus is occurring. Take notes of your observations. For example, ABC notes for the grocery store meltdowns exemplified above, might look like the following:

Finally, carefully consider what small changes you can make before your child's behavior of focus typically occurs (antecedent interventions) and how you can respond differently after the behavior of focus occurs (consequence interventions).

TABLE 5.1 Example of ABC Data Collection

Antecedent	Behavior	Consequence
• I told Lucy to put the cereal box back on the shelf	• Lucy threw herself on the floor of the cereal aisle in tears	• I said "I don't like how you are acting right now" and put the cereal box in the basket
• I pushed the cereal box aside at checkout	• Lucy dropped to the floor/ crying hard and loud	• I put the box onto the conveyer belt and apologized to the clerk

Ask yourself the following questions to inform possible antecedent interventions:

◆ Can I provide choice before making a request/stating a demand? ("It is time to get ready for bed, do you want to wear the Paw Patrol PJ or Spider Man PJ?")

◆ Can I change who is present or when a routine takes place? (Can a novel caregiver initiate bedtime or can bath precede dinner?)

◆ Can I give my child a "head's up" prior to a difficult transition? ("Five minutes and then it is time to put PJs on.")

◆ Can I use a visual support/cue in place of a verbal request? (Visual schedule of bedtime routine, a photo of what being ready for bed looks like.)

◆ Can I make an environment more sensory-friendly for my child before entering it? (Can lighting/noise level be reduced/blocked?)

◆ Can I give my child a lot of attention, before an attention-seeking problem behavior is likely to happen? (Fifteen minutes of 1:1 play, before making a work call.)

Ask yourself the following questions to inform possible consequence interventions:

◆ Can I "catch my child being good" to quickly reinforce and strengthen desired behaviors that occur naturally?

◆ Can I use if/then statements to quickly redirect an undesired behavior? ("If you sit in your chair, then I will bring you your juice.")

◆ Can I use a verbal/nonverbal cue to quickly redirect an undesired behavior by reminding my child to use the previously taught replacement behavior? ("If you are upset you can say.")
◆ Can I use a token economy for my child to earn preferred items/activities only after engaging in desired behaviors (sticker chart, coin chart)?

Before you begin your own ABC analysis, remember that if you have not worked on your child's behavior in a while, it is expected to initially worsen before improving. Think of a baby being trained to fall asleep on its own. Crying often increases before it settles down. Be sure your behavior of focus is one that you can safely and consistently address before attempting to change your child's behavior by changing your own. Ask yourself:

◆ Can I safely and consistently ignore a behavior that is reinforced by attention?
◆ Can I safely and proactively provide breaks from challenging environments/situations to avoid behavior that is maintained by escape?

When to Get Help

Your family's safety, health, and overall well-being are of highest priority when determining a course of action to address behavior change. Ask yourself the following questions when considering whether to partner with ABA service providers. If you answer yes to one or more, you are encouraged to seek support.

Do any behaviors pose a risk of harm to my child or others?

◆ Aggression (causing physical harm to another with intention)
◆ Self-injury (causing physical harm to oneself with intention)
◆ Wandering/elopement (moving away or towards something without supervision)
◆ Noncompliance to safety precautions (refusing/escaping car seat/belt)

Do any behaviors interfere with daily health or safety for my child or our family?

♦ Wandering or elopement (running away or towards something without supervision)
♦ Feeding (extreme food selectivity/refusal)
♦ Sleeping (poor sleep hygiene, sleep avoidance/frequent night waking)
♦ Toileting (delayed, inconsistent, resistant)
♦ Self-care (refusing medication, resistant to hygiene routines)

Do any behaviors prevent our family from participating in social events/activities?

♦ Avoiding family gatherings (celebrations, dinners)
♦ Excessive absenteeism (school avoidance, tardiness)
♦ Avoiding participating in leisure activities in the community (eating in restaurants)
♦ Avoiding existing social support networks (faith-based services)

It is our hope that your family has access to high quality ABA services. However, you may need do a little research to find a service provider that is the best fit for you and your child. You can start by posing the following questions to providers:

♦ How many BCBAs do you have on staff?
♦ Does you have a BCBA with specialized training/expertise in _____?
♦ Where will services be provided?
♦ Will I be provided with training/support?
♦ How and when will my child's progress be communicated to me?

Summary

You can learn a lot about what your child is trying to communicate by taking a closer and more objective look at problem behavior when it occurs. Understanding ABA principles and strategies can help you feel more prepared to plan for and address your child's challenging behaviors. The strategies provided here can also help you teach your child better ways to communicate their needs and frustrations. Some behaviors can be successfully addressed by you in the home. Others will need the support of professionals. Together, you can prevent or minimize problem behaviors and promote functional and effective communication for your child.

Resources

Association for Science in Autism Treatment: Early Intensive Behavior Intervention

> https://asatonline.org/for-parents/learn-more-about-spe-
> cific-treatments/early-intensive-behavioral-interventiontre
> atment-2/
> Behavior Analyst Certification Board
> https://www.bacb.com/
> Parent Training for Disruptive Behavior: The RUBI Autism
> Network https://www.rubinetwork.org/
> The Big Red Safety Tool Kit
> https://asatonline.org/research-treatment/resources/topical
> -articles/big-red-safety-tool-kit/

References

Baer, D. M., Wolf, M. M., & Risley, T. R. (1968). Some current dimensions of applied behavior analysis. *Journal of Applied Behavior Analysis*, *1*(1), 91–97.

Foxx, R. M. (2008). Applied behavior analysis treatment of autism: The state of the art. *Child and adolescent psychiatric clinics of North America*, *17*(4), 821–834.

6

Speech and Language Therapy

Speech and Language Therapy Explained

Although communication abilities vary greatly from child to child, all children with autism will have some speech, language, or social communication deficits that require focused intervention (see Chapter 1). Some children may not be able to speak using verbal language. Others will have limited vocabulary and/ or limited interests that make it difficult to maintain conversations. Some may have very advanced language skills and shared interests, but still struggle to understand others or to be understood in daily social interactions.

For this reason, no matter what your child's level of need is at the time of diagnosis, speech and language therapy is likely the first line of intervention to consider. It is highly recommended that speech and language therapy begin as early as possible and that it remains a prioritized intervention for your child. Your child may need therapy just for speech or just for language, or both. The distinction between the two is described below:

- ♦ **Speech:** How sounds are spoken through articulation (using lips, mouth, and tongue muscles), voice (volume, pitch), and fluency (the rhythm of speech)
- ♦ **Language:** How words are used to communicate fluently

DOI: 10.4324/9781003285953-7

Your child may also need therapy just for expressive language deficits, or just for receptive language deficits, or both. The distinction between the two is described below:

- **Expressive language:** How well your child uses verbal and/or nonverbal language to communicate with others
- **Receptive language:** How well your child understands the verbal and/or nonverbal language communicated by others

The most important goal for *all* children with autism is to ensure they can communicate effectively. They must be able to use language functionally to get their needs met and to advocate for themselves. They must also be able to use language socially to establish and maintain relationships and be meaningfully included in home, community, school, work, and leisure settings. Therefore, it is also necessary to think about your child's language development in the following terms:

- **Functional communication:** The ability to spontaneously and independently use language to communicate wants and needs
- **Social pragmatics:** The ability to use language socially, change language based on social context, and follow social norms during social interactions

If your child does not have a reliable mode of communication that achieves both functional and social communication goals, then they may benefit from the use of Augmentative and Alternative Communication (ACC). ACC is nonverbal communication forms that can be used with or without assistance and in conjunction with the development of verbal language when appropriate. Some examples are:

- Sign language
- Picture exchange systems
- iPad and similar speech generation devices
- Text-to-speech software.

Your child's unique abilities, challenges, and preferences should be considered when making communication-related decisions with and for them. It is not enough for your child to be understood in your home or in the clinic where receiving speech and language services. They must be empowered to use their "voice" with the people that are most important to them and in the places they spend most of their time, now and in the future.

Speech and Language Services

Communication-related services are provided in the home, community, clinics, and schools. Services may be offered through early intervention programs (ages 0–3) or special education programs (ages 3–22) for children who are eligible for these services. They are also offered privately and can be accessed through some insurance plans and/or private pay. All members of your child's support team should be addressing communication goals in collaboration with you and one another, as this is the primary area of need for children with autism. However, there are two types of professionals who have more specialized training and can help you make important communication-related decisions. Although they approach language differently, they share the same goals.

Speech and Language Pathologist (SLP)

The SLP is a trained and credentialed professional who addresses speech and language disorders and a wide range of social communication goals. They may also address academic goals related to communication, such as reading comprehension and/or written expression. Some SLPs also specialize in feeding and swallowing disorders. The SLP will begin by evaluating your child's abilities, developing appropriate goals, and determining an intervention plan. The American Speech, Language and Hearing Association (ASHA) has a list of qualified providers.

Board Certified Behavior Analyst (BCBA)

Providers who practice Applied Behavior Analysis (ABA) are also an essential part of your child's speech and language team. Especially when the focus is to develop functional language and social interaction skills for your child. A BCBA will approach language development using the following evidenced-based methods:

◆ **Functional communication training (FCT):** As discussed in Chapter 5, problem behavior is a form of communication. For children who do not have advanced language skills, it may be the only means of communicating their wants, needs, and feelings. FCT replaces problem behavior with a more common and socially appropriate form of communication that serves the same function. Extinction, or ending reinforcement for the problem behavior, is used in conjunction with immediate reinforcement for the replacement communication. This can include verbal and nonverbal language as well as ACC when necessary

◆ **Verbal behavior (VB):** This approach teaches language and communication by connecting words to the purpose they serve. The goal is to show children that communication serves an important function in their daily life. The child learns that words get them access to desired items or activities and help them avoid aversive ones. Rather than focusing on how to say words, VB teaches why and when they should be used. This approach classifies language into four categories:

◆ **Mands:** Words used to make requests

◆ **Tacts:** Words used to label or draw shared attention to a single object, person, etc.

◆ **Intraverbals:** Words used to interact with others

◆ **Echoics:** Repeated words

The VB approach begins with mands, as this is the most socially motivating for children and shows immediately that communication serves a function for them. This approach is best when it is integrated in the child's natural environment so they can see how requests can be met by the people they see every day.

As discussed in Chapter 12, your child might have an Individualized Family Service Plan (IFSP) or an Individualized Education Program (IEP) that will target speech and language goals that are specific to your child's needs. The IEP will also spell out what methods will be used to address them. Sample speech and language goals might include (see Chapter 12 for how these should be stated in observable and measurable terms):

◆ The child will produce a variety of speech sounds
◆ The child will use a range of gestures to communicate (e.g., pointing, nodding)
◆ The child will respond accurately to "wh" questions (who, what, where, when)
◆ The child will use picture cues to identify the emotion of characters in a story
◆ The child will make a request (mand) for a desired item or activity without prompting
◆ The child will be able to label (tact) people and/or items in the classroom

What the Research Reports

The National Professional Development Center (NPDC) on Autism Spectrum Disorder identified Augmentative and Alternative Communication (AAC) and Functional Communication Training (FCT) as evidence-based practices for children, youths, and young adults with autism. In 2020, this comprehensive report noted the following positive outcomes related to effective communication. A number of studies report similar positive findings (Battaglia, 2017; Gantz et al., 2011; Still et al., 2014).

AAC

◆ Pre-academic and academic skills for children to youth (birth to 14)
◆ Play skills for children to youth (birth to 14)
◆ Challenging/interfering behaviors for children to youth (birth to 14)
◆ Pre-academic and academic skills for children to youth (birth to 14)

- Communication skills for children to young adults (birth to 22)
- Social skills for children to young adults (birth to 22)

FCT

- Adaptive/self-help skills for children to young adults (birth to 22)
- Play skills for children to youth (birth to 14)
- Challenging/interfering behaviors for children to youth (birth to 14)
- Communication skills for children to young adults (birth to 22)
- School readiness skills for children to youth (birth to 14)
- Social skills for children to young adults (birth to 22)

Verbal Behavior (VB)

In 2006, Sauter and LeBlanc conducted a review of the literature on the VB approach and reported that 60 articles published in 11 well-respected journals concluded that it was effective in developing functional and social language skills for individuals with autism. There is a large body of evidence to support this to date. However, there is not as much evidence that the benefits of this approach extend to the other communication-related skill domains listed above.

A Cautionary Report

As stated emphatically in a 2018 article by Ganz and colleagues, there is no evidence that "facilitated communication" (supported typing where an adult guides a child's hands to produce language) is verifiable or effective. Furthermore, it has been reported that this highly discredited approach contributes to issues related to safety and exploitation and other "dire results" (Gantz et al., 2018). This has been a source of a number of lawsuits initiated by parents on behalf of their children and young adults with autism. There has been a recent resurgence of this approach in the media and other unreliable outlets, so be aware of the science discrediting it again and again. See the ASHA position statement on this: https://www.asha.org/policy/ps2018-00352/.

Quick Start to Using Speech and Language Therapy

Remember the goal of communication is both functional and social. Embed communication supports into naturally occurring daily activities as much as possible. Start by helping your child make requests for their favorite things (e.g., juice, goldfish, iPad, etc.), as this is the most motivating and easiest to reinforce quickly. This is also true for protesting non-preferred items or activities (e.g., saying no, requesting space or a break). Saying no is a healthy developmental milestone for young children, and children with autism also have the right to this autonomy (within reason). However, they need to do it safely and appropriately.

Recognize each problem behavior as a communication attempt. Identify a verbal or nonverbal replacement for it that serves the same function. Keep it as simple as possible. Replacement communication should require less, not more effort than the problem behavior. Reinforce the use of the replacement communication immediately by honoring the request or protest. The immediate responding can later be faded out to become more natural, but at first you are keeping a strict contract with your child. For example, "First use your new word we practiced (verbal or nonverbal), then you get X" (your need or want will be met immediately).

Talk to your child a lot every day. Narrate your thoughts and actions as you go about your daily routines when possible. They are listening and learning. An exception is when your child is very upset or frustrated as then you only need to use a few supportive and directive words. You interact with your child every day so identify some time to work towards social communication goals together. Keep it positive and fun. They will learn from you without knowing they are doing hard work. Try the following.

Prompting

- ◆ Create communication temptations (e.g., place a desired item just out of reach and prompt requesting the previously taught word, verbal or nonverbal)

- Use choice boards (e.g., pictures of snacks or items chosen verbally or nonverbally)
- Create "break cards" for your child to use to communicate frustration or the need to temporarily escape a demand
- Point to items for your child to label (tact) during daily tasks (e.g., child can name items while grocery shopping). If they are able, switch roles

Reinforcement

- Reinforce new attempts to make requests/protests appropriately by responding quickly
- Reinforce new attempts to gain your attention appropriately by responding quickly
- Reinforce turn taking, waiting turn to speak
- Reinforce approximations/attempts to use practiced words (verbal or nonverbal) even if they are not exact, then provide feedback to shape response

Reading

- Build vocabulary during shared reading (pause to ask who, what, where questions)
- Build language comprehension during shared reading (pause to ask why, how questions)
- Expand language during shared reading (have your child repeat adjectives, attributes you use to describe objects or characters in the book, etc.)
- Think aloud during shared reading (wonder out loud to model thinking about the story)
- Have your child predict what might happen next in a story
- Pause and prompt your child to make inferences about how a character is feeling and why by attending to picture cues
- Help your child to make text-to-life connections (relate story to an event in their life)

Playing

- ◆ Play question games (hide a familiar item in a bag and model asking questions to guess what it is)
- ◆ Play copy the gesture (have your child imitate your gestures and respond to them as would be expected of them)
- ◆ Play label the facial expression (role play, picture cards, or in stories)
- ◆ Play match the emotion to facial expression or a causal situation
- ◆ Play sorting and matching games with like words or concepts
- ◆ Play turn-taking games with the goal of praising appropriate waiting
- ◆ Play eye-spy with the goal of supporting vocabulary and joint attention

Summary

Early intervention is key, as speech and language skills are developed and shaped over time. Establishing a reliable mode of communication for your child, verbally or nonverbally, should be the prioritized goal of any intervention plan. The best way to get communication started is to teach your child that it serves an immediate and desirable function. The best way to develop social communication skills is to address these skills as naturally as possible by embedding evidence-based strategies into your child's natural environment and with the people they interact with the most.

If you do not have professional speech and language services yet, inquire about how to access this in your child's school and/or through private services. Stay an active participant in these services and help your child to generalize the skills learned in therapy to their everyday lives. Choose one or two of the activities previously suggested and get started today.

Resources

American Speech Language Hearing Association (ASHA)
https://www.asha.org/
Social Thinking®
https://www.socialthinking.com/
The Program for the Education and Enrichment of Relational
  Skills (PEERS®)
https://www.semel.ucla.edu/peers

References

Battaglia, D. (2017). Functional communication training in children with autism spectrum disorder. *Young Exceptional Children, 20*(1), 30–40. https://doi.org/10.1177/1096250615576809.

Ganz, J. B., Earles-Vollrath, T. L., Heath, A. K., Parker, R. I., Rispoli, M. J., & Duran, J. B. (2011). A meta-analysis of single case research studies on aided augmentative and alternative communication systems with individuals with autism spectrum disorders. *Journal of Autism and Developmental Disorders, 42*(1), 60–74. https://doi.org/10.1007/s10803-011-1212-2.

Ganz, J. B., Katsiyannis, A., & Morin, K. L. (2018). Facilitated communication: The resurgence of a disproven treatment for individuals with autism. *Intervention in School and Clinic, 54*(1), 52–56. https://doi.org/10.1177/1053451217692564.

Still, K., Rehfeldt, R. A., Whelan, R., May, R., & Dymond, S. (2014). Facilitating requesting skills using high-tech augmentative and alternative communication devices with individuals with autism spectrum disorders: A systematic review. *Research in Autism Spectrum Disorders, 8*(9), 1184–1199. https://doi.org/10.1016/j.rasd.2014.06.003.

7

Occupational Therapy

Occupational Therapy Explained

Occupational therapy (OT) is a holistic intervention that focuses on helping individuals with autism successfully participate in daily activities (occupations) and use everyday objects (e.g., writing, feeding utensils, etc.). The overarching goal of OT is to promote independence and well-being across the life span. OT helps with any needs related to play, school, or work. Rather than focusing on a single developmental domain, OT considers the strengths and limitations of the whole child and aims to eliminate any barriers that prevent them from fully participating in daily living activities across settings. Most commonly, OT addresses the following broad domains:

- ◆ Sensory modulation
- ◆ Motor skills
- ◆ Cognitive skills
- ◆ Social participation
- ◆ Communication skills
- ◆ Daily living skills

The American Occupational Therapy Association (AOTA), the largest national professional organization, identified the following as OT interventions that you can expect for different ages:

DOI: 10.4324/9781003285953-8

- Daily living skills training
- Motor development and planning skills
- Sensory integration strategy development
- Social-emotional strategy development
- Peer-mediated strategies
- Play and/or leisure participation
- Self-advocacy skills training
- Transitioning to adulthood
- Work/employment skills

Occupational Therapy Services

OT services are provided through early intervention programs (ages 0–3) or special education programs (ages 3–21) for children who are found eligible for these services. They are also offered privately and can be accessed through some insurance plans and/or private pay. Services are delivered both in natural environments (home, community, schools) and in clinical settings by occupational therapists licensed by the National Board for Certification in Occupational Therapy, or NBCOT. Services might also be delivered by a Certified Occupational Therapy Assistant (COTA) under the supervision of the Masters Level Occupational Therapist. To locate qualified providers, you can visit https://www.nbcot.org/

Most often, occupational therapists work as part of an interdisciplinary team with the shared goal of promoting early detection and intervention for developmental delays through collaborative and family-focused care (e.g., speech therapists, physical therapists, behavior analysts, educators). OT will begin with a comprehensive assessment of your child to determine their current level of ability and independence in daily living skills.

The therapist will also identify any gaps between what your child can do now and what they will be expected to do in a given play, school, or work environment. Most commonly, occupational therapists target the following daily activities for children with autism:

- Dressing routines
- Feeding behaviors

◆ Grooming behaviors
◆ Toileting
◆ Handwriting
◆ Coloring
◆ Cutting with scissors
◆ Initiating play
◆ Asking for help
◆ Tolerating/avoiding sensory discomfort

As discussed in Chapter 12, your child might have an Individualized Family Service Plan or an Individualized Education Program that will target OT goals that are specific to your child's strengths and limitations. Sample OT goals might include (see Chapter 12 for how these should be stated in observable and measurable terms):

◆ The child will pick up small objects using a pincer grasp
◆ The child will write lower case letters in good formation
◆ The child will cut across a piece of paper in a straight line
◆ The child will complete interlocking puzzles
◆ The child will stack a specified numbers of blocks
◆ The child will complete grooming tasks with increasing independence
◆ The child will complete a toileting routine with a specified level of independence
◆ The child will tolerate oral hygiene for a specified amount of time
◆ The child will tolerate standing in line for a specified amount of time
◆ The child will tolerate sitting in their designated space during circle time
◆ The child will initiate play with a same-aged peer

What the Research Reports

In 2008, Case-Smith and Arbesman conducted a systematic review of the research describing OT-related interventions for individuals with autism. The study was conducted in collaboration with AOTA as part of a broader "Evidence-Based Literature Review" project. Although the researchers examined six broad areas in this study, they identified three as the one most commonly addressed by Occupational Therapists alone or as part of team-based care. They reported the following findings on each.

Sensory Integration and Sensory-Based Interventions

The researchers categorized this broad approach into three commonly used interventions: sensory integration training, sensory-based interventions, and auditory integration training. It was noted that despite the specialized knowledge and experience occupational therapists have in sensory-based interventions such as these, there is limited empirical support for their use with children with autism or their efficacy in developing specific skills.

Within the small evidence base available, there were some positive effects on behavior modulation and social participation reported. Of these, massaging interventions had the most notable promise for reducing hyperactivity, impulsivity, and stereotypical behaviors in children with autism. Auditory integration training had the weakest support. It was concluded that sensory-focused interventions are best when part of a comprehensive package and that they should be paired with more functional skill-building interventions.

Relationship-Based, Interactive Interventions

Interventions that incorporate imitation (adult imitating child's actions), positive responding, prompting, and facilitated peer interactions were identified as the most impactful for increasing the social engagement of children with autism participating in social/play-focused interventions. It was also noted that structured play activities, especially those that include prompting and reinforcement, have had positive effects on turn-taking, sharing, communication, and social interaction. Results were enhanced when activities used high interest play materials, with a special mention of Legos™.

Developmental Skill-Based Programs

Programs that used developmentally appropriate play-based approaches and emphasize positive affect, nonverbal communication, social relationships, and classroom structure were reported to have positive effects on children with autism's cognition, communication, and social-emotional skills. Those that incorporate visual cueing and environmental modifications were noted to have some enhanced effect on communication. However, the research on this is limited and the results were inconclusive.

Sensory Integration®

In their 2021 report, The National Professional Development Center (NPDC) identified Sensory Integration as an evidence-based practice for individuals with autism for the first time. However, they specify that the evidence base for Sensory Integration is explicit in the approach developed by Jean Ayres (2005). Other stand-alone sensory-based interventions (i.e., auditory integration, sensory diets) are not considered to be research-based approaches, despite their popularity and continued use in practice (Steinbrenner et al., 2020, Wong et al., 2015).

Parents' Perceptions of Sensory-Based Interventions (SBIs)

In 2019, Peña and colleagues reported on the efficacy of SBIs to address challenging behaviors in children with autism from the parents' perspective. The researchers noted here that there is limited research supporting the use of SBIs for this specific purpose. Parents reported Occupational Therapists most commonly recommended the use of trampolines, massage, and oral-motor tools. In order of frequency, parents reported that the most used interventions in the home were massage, trampoline, joint compressions, and brushing techniques. Based on parents' survey responses, more than half believed that SBIs had positive effects on their children's challenging behavior. However, they noted that the interventions were difficult to use on their own and that they had limited access to appropriate materials.

Quick Start to Using Occupational Therapy

Your child may benefit from the holistic and comprehensive expertise of an occupational therapist. The family-focused approach commonly utilized by these professionals can help you better identify what developmental goals should be addressed and for what purposes. Find out what OT services are available for your child and who is best to deliver them and where, based on your child's unique areas of need.

There are also a number of developmentally and parent-friendly activities that can be done in your home to support your child's OT-related needs without assistance. Choose engaging play-based activities that are also skill-building. Below are a few examples of some play activities that support a range of developmental skills.

Fine Motor

- ◆ Sort small items such as colored beads into colored bins
- ◆ Play with interlocking blocks (Legos™)
- ◆ Play with finger puppets
- ◆ Cut out different shapes to make a picture or collage
- ◆ Use cookie cutters with playdough
- ◆ Use stencils to support writing
- ◆ Use lacing boards or similar toys

Gross Motor

- ◆ Use trampolines for balance
- ◆ Play hopscotch for coordination
- ◆ Climb playground structures for motor planning
- ◆ Ride tricycles, bicycles, or scooters to support all of the above
- ◆ Use dancing games and programs to support all of the above
- ◆ Do different "animal walks"

Sensory

♦ Create a fidget tool kit with safe and engaging small items
♦ Blow bubbles
♦ Play toy instrument (recorder, harmonica)
♦ Play with sand tables and toys
♦ Pay with water tables and toys
♦ Use finger paints
♦ Draw picture in shaving cream

Social Participation

♦ Play turn taking games
♦ Play role, pass, or throw the ball to (name)
♦ Play Simon Says
♦ Play Follow the Leader
♦ Play pretend or fantasy games
♦ Play games that are common to your child's age and teach social rules (e.g., tag)
♦ Use your child's special interest to increase motivation to participate in shared play

Summary

The goal of OT is to increase your child's ability to participate as fully and independently in daily activities (occupations) as possible. The skills required to do so are broad, and therefore the approaches used to address these skills are often comprehensive and holistic in nature. They are also best addressed in natural environments, so children can learn the play and work skills they need to be successful and meaningfully included in these settings. Team-based approaches are also beneficial, as expertise in communication, motor planning, sensory modulation, and behavior modification is often required to teach skills that can be maintained over time and generalized to different settings.

Your role in this is an important one. If you are benefiting from an occupational therapist as part of your support team, learn from them. Find time to introduce the play-based activities shared here to develop a variety of skills during everyday routines. Have fun doing them. Feel confident knowing that play is the work of children and the quality time you spend playing with your child is time well spent for both of you.

Resources

American Occupational Therapy Association: Fact Sheets
https://www.aota.org/about-occupational-therapy/professionals/master-list.aspx
American Occupational Therapy Association: State Contact Information
https://myaota.aota.org/asapcontacts.aspx?_ga=2.48667235.45743269.1579114130-1501816344.1579114130

References

Ayres, A. J., & Robbins, J. (2005). *Sensory integration and the child: Understanding hidden sensory challenges.* Los Angels, CA: Western psychological services.

Steinbrenner, J. R., Hume, K., Odom, S. L., Morin, K. L., Nowell, S. W., Tomaszewski, B., ... & Savage, M. N. (2020). *Evidence-based practices for children, youth, and young adults with autism.* Chapel Hill, NC: FPG Child Development Institute.

Wong, C., Odom, S. L., Hume, K. A., Cox, A. W., Fettig, A., Kucharczyk, S., ... & Schultz, T. R. (2015). Evidence-based practices for children, youth, and young adults with autism spectrum disorder: A comprehensive review. *Journal of Autism and Developmental Disorders, 45*(7), 1951–1966.

8

Physical Therapy and Exercise

Physical Therapy and Exercise Explained

Pediatric physical therapy involves activities and exercises that build your child's gross motor skills and help strengthen muscles and improve motor control. Interestingly, while most children with autism have motor deficits, a motor deficit is not a core autism symptom. The only motor deficit included in the diagnostic criteria for autism is the presence of repetitive behaviors. However, motor deficits in children with autism are increasingly being recognized and supported so physical therapists have expanded their role in the treatment of children with autism.

Physical therapy is not a lifelong support so your child might need physical therapy the most when he or she is young and then at various other times during his or her development. Physical therapists work with children starting at birth and the range of their supports is customized to meet your child's needs. Since each child's challenges and goals are different, a physical therapist designs a program to specifically help your child. Physical therapists may work with very young children on basic motor skills such as sitting, rolling, standing, walking, and imitating. Older children might work on skills such as kicking, using school bus stairs, carrying materials, and eye-hand coordination with throwing and catching. These skills promote physical and social growth.

DOI: 10.4324/9781003285953-9

Physical therapy can also address your child's sensory issues. The physical therapist may utilize brushing, massage, deep touching, swings, spinning, or weighted vests. These activities can help your child learn to cope with sensory information. Your child's physical therapists may collaborate with your child's behavior therapist as well.

A physical therapist works in hospitals, clinics, private practice, and schools. Thus, some children receive physical therapy during the school day as well as outside of school in a clinic or center. Your child's physical therapist will consult with you about your child's progress as well as help you learn activities to support your child. Many therapists encourage parents to watch or become involved in therapy sessions in order to continue therapy at home. This consistency will improve your child's strength, balance, coordination.

We recommend you work with a certified physical therapist who has experience working with children with autism. Your insurance or pediatrician can often be able to provide a list of pediatric physical therapists. In addition, your child's school might provide physical therapy services through their employees. The American Physical Therapy Association also has a list of providers.

When a physical therapist begins working with your child, you should expect:

- ◆ Evaluation of your child's abilities such as:
- ◆ Posture strength
- ◆ Coordination
- ◆ Hopping, jumping, running
- ◆ Positioning when sitting on furniture
- ◆ Body awareness
- ◆ Play skills
- ◆ Behavior
- ◆ Ability to make transitions
- ◆ Preferred toys or play themes
- ◆ Understating safety statements such as "stop"
- ◆ Observing your child
- ◆ Talking with you about your goals for your child
- ◆ Writing a specific treatment plan for your child

As discussed in Chapter 12, your child might have an Individualized Education Program (IEP). Sample IEP physical therapy goals might include:

- The child will build arm, balance, and core strength by sitting/ balancing on therapy ball for 1 minute on three out of four trials
- The child will increase arm strength by holding therapy ball in four posture holds for 30 seconds on three out of four trials
- The child will initiate three steps independently to reach desired reinforcer
- The child will walk from classroom to bathroom with facilitation at shoulders, without stopping one time per school day
- The child, while standing, will squat to retrieve a tray and ten letter magnets from the floor and return to standing three consecutive times

While many children receive support from a physical therapist, it's equally important for your child to engage in physical activities for play and leisure time. Yet, as important as exercise is, it's usually not a preferred activity of children with autism. As a parent you understand, and research has identified, children with autism have many barriers to physical activity including:

- Sensory issues
- Social anxiety
- Medication effects
- Metabolic abnormalities
- Sleep disturbances
- Atypical eating patterns
- Low intellectual ability
- Lack of knowledge or awareness about exercise benefits
- Behavioral problems
- Motor skills deficits
- Parental time constraints
- A lack of opportunities

Furthermore, children with autism are at risk for poor motor coordination, core strength, posture, and balance. Nevertheless, kids with autism benefit from physical play and exercise. Benefits of exercise for children with autism include:

◆ Reduction in problem behaviors
◆ Fewer stereotypical behaviors
◆ Less hyperactivity
◆ Reduce clumsiness
◆ Less self-injurious behavior
◆ Improve emotional regulation
◆ Increase body and spatial awareness
◆ Increase focus

Exercise also contributes to healthy living, stimulates the digestive system, and can help the brain release positive endorphins.

Younger children with autism are more physically active than older children and participate in exercise modalities including walking, jogging, swimming, bicycling, playing cornhole, roller skating, horseback riding, and using exergames. Your child benefits from any physical activity regardless of if it occurs in school, home, or outpatient clinic. Family involvement in exercising together also increases motivation and improves exercise outcomes.

What the Research Reports

Research on physical therapy benefits was limited and research often focused on physical activity benefits for children with autism. Research thoroughly documented concerns about motor impairments and children with autism. Hilton and colleagues (2012) reported that up to 83% of children with autism spectrum disorder have difficulty performing age-appropriate motor skills. These motor impairments contribute to a child being overweight, being more sedentary, and finding less enjoyment in physical activity.

Rebecca Downey and colleagues (2012) completed a complete review of research literature and concluded there was impaired motor activity in children who have the diagnosis of autism. They stated, "Although impaired motor activity is not included in the diagnosis, impaired motor activity appears to be an observable trend" (p. 7).

Although children with autism have motor impairments, these impairments can be improved. Exercise and Movement was one evidenced-based intervention noted in the 2020 Evidenced-Based Practices for Children, Youth, and Young Adults with Autism report as discussed in Chapter 2. As noted on page 82 of the report, "Exercise can be used as an antecedent activity to improve performance in a task or behavior, or it can be used to increase physical fitness and motor skills." A child's exercise and movement can be aerobic, strength, stretching, or skillful motor activities accomplished individually or in groups.

Ruggeri and colleagues (2020) reviewed studies with individuals with autism spectrum disorder ranging from the age of 3 to 19 years. They reported the motor abilities of children with ASD improved using various activities including gymnastics, soccer, throwing, catching, horse riding, swimming, video gaming, and physical education. They also reported children with autism understood instructions best visually, as compared to verbally.

Research presented by Menear and Neumeier (2015) suggested that, to prepare children with ASD for physical activities, readers use social narratives, prepare the environment to minimize sensory challenges, and adapt the activities to the child's motor development.

Based on research literature and Department of Health and Human Services guidelines, Srinivasan, Pescatello, and Bhat (2014) offered specific physical activity and exercise recommendations for children with ASD. They recommended at least three days per week of moderate aerobic exercise of 20–30 minutes per session. Types of aerobic exercise might include jogging, walk/run interval training, bicycling, swimming, treadmill training, and exergames such as Dance Dance Revolution by Nintendo™.

In addition, they recommended one day per week of resistance exercise. This would be one set of 6–15 reps. In children younger than ten years old, this might include jumping, climb-ing, or throwing. Children aged 10 and older could engage in a strengthening program for muscles using elastic bands, body weight resistance, or weight lifting machines with light resist-ance. Once to twice per week of flexibility and muscular train-ing was recommended. This could be up to an hour of muscle stretching, therapeutic horseback riding, aquatic exercises, yoga, or tai-chi.

In summary, this exercise program would include:

♦ Three days per week of 20–30 minute aerobic type exercise
♦ One day per week of resistance exercise including 6–15 repetitions
♦ One to two days per week of muscular training and flexibility

Quick Start to Using Physical Therapy and Exercise

You've heard the saying, "Success builds success" but unfortu-nately, many children with autism don't experience satisfying success when exercising. Their weak motor skills can limit par-ticipation in throwing, catching, bike riding, and gymnastics. Their sensory processing differences such as tactile hypersensi-tivity might interfere with participation. Given these challenges, we want to choose and structure our kids' activities that lead to success and enjoyment. We all like doing things we are good at, and we often repeat them.

Three key components for helping your child exercise are to:

♦ Provide visual directions (pictures, videos, or demonstrations)
♦ Use social narratives
♦ Prepare the environment to minimize sensory challenges
♦ And adapt the activities, if needed

There are no autism-specific physical therapy activities or exer-cises. This implies there is a wide-open playing field for you to choose exercise activities for your child. If your child resists exercise, sometimes you can pair exercise with a known reinforcer. Thus, if kicking a ball is not a preferred task, he might perform this nonpreferred task in order to get his preferred iPad time.

Exercising with your child can stimulate interest and involvement. Take a walk, swim in the pool, play cornhole, or dance together to your child's favorite song. Make it fun and laugh along the way. You might even find that your child's preferred reinforcer becomes spending time exercising with you.

Thus, success with exercising is more about engagement and enjoyment in the activity rather than having perfect form. Once your child enjoys exercising you can refine form and posture. Below you'll find some exercises and activities often completed in physical therapy sessions.

◆ Ball bounce. In this activity, the child uses a medium-sized inflatable ball and tosses it against a wall. As the ball comes off the wall, practice catching the ball using two hands, one hand, or using a Velcro glove

◆ Balancing. Your child might first balance on one foot, then the other. As your child becomes more proficient, time her to see how long she can stay on one foot. Some children like to try and beat their time

◆ Soccer ball. Your child might stop the ball, position it, and pass it back

◆ Crossing arms. Your child will cross arms by making them into an X across his chest with the left hand resting on the right shoulder and the right hand resting on the left shoulder. He then extends his hands up into the air and then straight out to the sides. While his hands are extended out to the sides, rotate them five times forward followed by five times backward

◆ Jumping in place. Your child jumps in place. Variations can include jumping with hands extended forward or hands extended to the side. Jump with one foot at a time or jump using both feet

- Heel to toe walking. Use colored painter's tape to tape a line on carpet. Your child practices walking placing one foot in front of the other in a heel to toe pattern
- Balancing board. You can make or purchase a balance board and your child can stand on the balancing board with assistance. Gradually reduce your support as your child becomes better at balancing
- Jump rope. It's a classic activity involving coordination and cardio
- Standing push-ups. Your child stands up and extends arms, slightly leans forward against a latched door or wall, and does standing push-ups
- Superman. Your child lies on the floor on her belly. Her arms are extended out in front of her. She can try to do superman by slightly lifting her arms and legs up off the floor at the same time
- Bear crawl. Your child should place feet and hands on the floor as if standing like a bear. Next, extend legs until slightly bent, walk from point A to B using feet and hands to move. Place palms on the floor and spread fingers wide like a bear claw
- Crossover march. Your child slowly marches in place. As he lifts his right knee up, he touches it with his left hand. As he lifts his left knee up, he touches it with his right hand

Leisure time activities might include:

- Use your child's Nintendo Switch™ and have exergaming exercise with video game play
- Jump rope, do jumping jacks, or burpee and set a personal best record. Each time try to beat your record
- Watch the television show American Ninja Warrior and create a small home course
- Jump on a trampoline
- If available, participate in a local exercise program such as "cross fit for kids"

- ◆ Play the game Twister. This helps with movement and following directions
- ◆ Listen to music and dance. For example, play the song from the Disney movie Madagascar, "I Like to Move It Move It" and have a dance party
- ◆ Train for and participate in the Special Olympics
- ◆ Bike ride
- ◆ Go for a brisk walk

Summary

Exercising might not be your child's favorite activity but there are tremendous benefits from exercising ranging from less hyperactivity, fewer stereotypical behaviors, increasing metabolism, improving strength, and releasing positive endorphins. You might need to use behavioral principles such as exercise to earn a preferred activity. Some children work better for someone other than a parent so he or she might exercise more with a physical therapist or coach. Keep in mind the fun principle and try to make exercising fun using music or exergaming with your child. It is alright to start small. Three minutes of exercising today is better than zero minutes yesterday.

Resources

American Physical Therapy Association
https://www.apta.org
Pediatric Physical Therapy Activities with Amy Sturkey, PT
https://youtu.be/NuvIuxTqyzw
Autism Exercise Specialist
https://www.autismexercisespecialist.com
Autism Fitness
https://autismfitness.com
15 Fun Fitness Activities for Kids
https://www.rasmussen.edu/degrees/education/blog/fun-fitness-activities-for-kids/

Chapter References

Downey, R., & Rapport, M. J. (2012). Motor activity in children with autism. *Pediatric Physical Therapy*, *24*(1), 2–20. https://doi.org/10.1097/PEP.0b013e31823db95f.

Hilton, C. L., Zhang, Y., Whilte, M. R., Klohr, C. L., & Constantino, J. (2012). Motor impairment in sibling pairs concordant and discordant for autism spectrum disorders. *Autism : The International Journal of Research and Practice*, *16*(4), 430–441. https://doi.org/10.1177/1362361311423018.

Menear, K. S., & Neumeier, W. H. (2015). Promoting physical activity for students with autism spectrum disorder: Barriers, benefits, and strategies for success. *Journal of Physical Education, Recreation and Dance, 86*(3), 43–48. https://doi.org/10.1080/07303084.2014.998395.

Ruggeri, A., Dancel, A., Johnson, R., & Sargent, B. (2020). The effect of motor and physical activity intervention on motor outcomes of children with autism spectrum disorder: A systematic review. *Autism*, *24*(3), 544–568. https://doi.org/10.1177/1362361319885215.

Srinivasan, S. M., Pescatello, L. S., & Bhat, A. N. (2014). Current perspectives on physical activity and exercise recommendations for children and adolescents with autism spectrum disorders. *Physical Therapy*, *94*(6), 875–889. https://doi.org/10.1080/07303084.2014.998395.

9

Cognitive Behavioral Therapy

Cognitive Behavioral Therapy Explained

Cognitive Behavioral Therapy (CBT) is used to treat a number of psychological and behavioral conditions that commonly occur in children with autism including:

- Generalized anxiety disorder
- Obsessive-compulsive disorder
- Attention deficit hyperactivity disorder
- Depression
- Insomnia

Since children with autism often experience more intense and persistent challenges related to these conditions early in life, CBT can be a very welcomed treatment with benefits for your whole family. The core principle of CBT is the premise that unhealthy thinking patterns can lead to unhealthy behavior patterns. The cyclical nature of this relationship is illustrated here.

CBT and applied behavioral analysis (ABA) draw upon the same principles and methods to address unhealthy behaviors common to autism and related mental health conditions. ABA addresses observable and measurable behaviors by identifying the environmental triggers that cause them to occur and the function they serve. CBT also targets observable and measurable behaviors in this way. However, CBT focuses on the cognitive

DOI: 10.4324/9781003285953-10

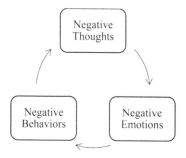

FIGURE 9.1 The Cyclical Nature of Unhealthy Thought Patterns

factors that cannot be observed (unhealthy, irrational, and obtrusive thoughts), but are known to serve as triggers for the unhelpful, and sometimes harmful, behaviors we can observe. To help you understand how the cognitive-behavioral cycle illustrated above can play out in the mind and body of a child, we will provide you with a "true-to-life" example.

A Case Study: Ana

Ana is a school-aged child diagnosed with autism and obsessive-compulsive disorder (OCD). OCD is a mental health condition characterized by obtrusive, repetitive, and irrational thoughts, followed by compulsive, excessive, and repetitive behaviors or rituals. Like autism, OCD presents differently from child to child and across time. For Ana right now, it presents as an intense fear of getting sick (especially vomiting) and greatly interferes with the quality of her day-to-day life. Ana has rituals she has to follow anytime she fears exposure to germs. She panics whenever she has to enter any situation that reminds her of vomiting. She avoids people, places, and things she associates with vomiting, even though they have no real correlation with the event (e.g., the clothes she wore, the place she sat, the movie she watched that day, etc.).

Like many children with autism, Ana has also been diagnosed with irritable bowel syndrome (IBS). Even though she is on a careful diet and her IBS does not result in vomiting, the abdominal discomfort she feels often triggers her irrational fear of vomiting and heightens her anxiety overall. In turn, the heightened anxiety often results in worsened digestive issues as she goes about her day. Her persistent anxiety and irrational fear of vomiting impact her eating, sleeping, social relationships, and school success in many ways. The table below exemplifies how the cognitive behavioral cycle plays out across a school day and the consequences Ana experiences from it.

The unwanted "what if" thoughts Ana has throughout the day do not relent unless she gives in to these unhelpful rituals. This cycle is exhausting and frustrating for both Ana and those who care for her on any given day. Ana is often unfairly reprimanded by the adults in her life and unnecessarily isolated from her peers. This is because her thoughts and emotions are not known to those around her, but her unusual, defiant, and seemingly unkind behavior is.

Ana's autism also makes it hard for her to process sensory information from her body accurately and prevents her from recognizing how her behaviors are interpreted by others. If people get angry at her, she does not have the perspective-taking skills to understand why or the social communication skills to advocate for herself differently.

There are a number of psychological and behavioral explanations on why this cycle is likely to continue without CBT. First, when Ana engages in the unhelpful coping behaviors, this brings her some temporary relief from the "what if" scenarios that circle through her head and the negative emotions that stem from them. However, each time these thoughts return, the negative emotions return. So, Ana feels compelled to repeat the same unhelpful behavior to experience the same temporary relief.

Second, these unhelpful behaviors are reinforced over time. Since Ana does not vomit in most instances as there was no real threat, she mistakenly correlates the unhelpful behaviors with the avoidance of vomiting. In other words, to Ana the threat was real each time and the rituals she followed were responsible for warding it off each time.

Third, once Ana's behaviors are reinforced in this way, they are very hard and sometimes even dangerous to redirect or interrupt. Stopping her from completing these routines can cause her great distress. If others don't comply with her requests to do the same, her anxiety turns to frustration and anger. This can result

TABLE 9.1 Daily Account of an Unhealthy Thought Emotion and Behavior Pattern

Unhealthy Thoughts	Unhealthy Emotions	Unhealthy Behaviors
At breakfast, Ana thinks... Last time I vomited, it was after eating eggs made the way they look on my plate right now, what if this happens again?	Ana feels... Fear and anxiety	To cope, Ana... • Refuses to sit in the same seat at the breakfast table that she sat in when she got sick last time and yells at her siblings until they switch with her, so they get mad at her • Refuses to eat anything at all at breakfast in case it touched the eggs, so she goes to school hungry • Pushes her parents away when they try to touch her after cooking eggs and yells at them to wash their hands again. She is late for school and her parents are late for work
At lunch, Ana thinks... I took a bite of a banana with brown marks on it, what if it makes me vomit when I get back to class?	Ana feels... Fear and anxiety	To cope, Ana... • Throws away her lunch after one bite of the banana even though she is still hungry from skipping breakfast • Makes frequent trips to the bathroom "just in case" she needs to vomit and misses out on instructions and work time • Ignores teachers when her name is called because her brain is "stuck" on these thoughts and gets repeatedly reprimanded • Avoids her friends so she does not vomit in front of them, and they get angry at her • Requests to go to the school nurse, and her parents are frustrated because they have to leave work to pick her up again
At bedtime, Ana thinks... Last time I vomited, it was in the middle of the night, what if I wake up in the night and have to vomit again?	Ana feels... Fear and anxiety	To cope, Ana... • Becomes aggressive to her parents when they try to make her comply with a bedtime routine • Refuses to sleep in her bed • Resists falling asleep to avoid waking up sick, so she and her parents are sleep deprived the next morning

in escalated behaviors such as aggression and self-harm. The temporary relief she feels when she engages in these coping rituals is way more reinforcing than anything her teachers, parents, or peers can offer or do in these moments.

Finally, Ana does not yet understand that her thoughts are automatic but can be changed or that thoughts can be irrational at times. She also does not yet have any replacement coping behaviors to do instead to deal with the negative emotions that result from them. This means we can only break the cycle by teaching a new one. CBT is the method for doing just that. The goal is to help children like Ana develop the cognitive awareness and self-regulation needed to identify unhealthy thoughts, tolerate uncomfortable emotions, and use healthy and effective coping strategies in response to them. CBT accomplishes this by treating both the unhealthy thinking patterns and the unhealthy behavior patterns simultaneously.

As children with autism vary in their cognitive, social, and emotional development, CBT may not be appropriate or well-timed for your child. However, there are a number of adapted approaches and intervention strategies that may be helpful for developing your child's emotional and self-regulation skills along the way. To help you decide if these approaches are right for your child now or in the future, it is helpful to know what the research says about who benefits most from them and when.

What the Research Reports

The research describes cognitive behavioral approaches in two ways:

1. Cognitive Behavioral Therapy (CBT)—a therapeutic approach delivered by a trained psychologist or related mental health professional in clinical sessions
2. Cognitive Behavioral Intervention Strategies (CBIS)—interventions for teaching learners how to evaluate their own thought and emotions and to self-regulate their own behavior with adult facilitation in more natural settings

This distinction is made here only to emphasize that the names of approaches and the people and settings who deliver them may change, but the core principles that are supported by psychological and behavioral research do not. The cognitive behavioral methods backed by research are those that systematically and simultaneously:

Address *unhealthy thinking patterns* by helping the learner:

♦ Understand thoughts are automatic but changeable
♦ Recognize distorted (irrational, unrealistic) or cata-strophic (worse-case scenario) thoughts
♦ Evaluate these thoughts in terms of reality (e.g., how true is…?, how likely is it…?)
♦ Reframe thoughts based on this evaluation (e.g., what is more likely?)
♦ Problem-solve situations based on this evaluation (e.g., If it is likely…, then I can…)
♦ Increase confidence in the ability to problem-solve over time (Last time, I was able to…)

Address *unhealthy behavior patterns* using some of the following methods:

♦ Cognitive restructuring: Replacing irrational thoughts with more balanced ones
♦ Containment: Setting parameters around when and where negative emotions and behaviors will be processed and addressed
♦ Graded exposure: Facing fearful situations in a gradual and therapeutic way over time
♦ Successive approximation: Breaking down complex tasks into smaller more attainable steps to build confidence and self-efficacy along the way

Cognitive Behavioral Therapy (CBT)

Research suggests that typically developing children are reported to benefit most from CBT beginning around the age of 7. A number of studies suggest that children with autism can also

benefit from CBT around this same developmental age when provided with some accommodations. In 2012, Lickel and colleagues
conducted a study for the purpose of assessing whether or not
children with autism between the ages of 7 and 12 have the prerequisite cognitive skills needed to successfully participate in
CBT-related tasks when compared to typically developing peers.

They identified emotion recognition, discrimination among
thoughts, feelings, and behaviors, and cognitive mediation as the
prerequisite skills needed for children to receive therapeutic benefits from this approach. The researchers found that, overall, children with autism performed as well as their typically developing
peers on CBT-related tasks. However, they noted that children
with autism struggled more with emotional recognition tasks
(identifying feelings and emotional states of others). The study
also suggests that older children and those with higher levels of
nonverbal intelligence may be the best candidates for CBT.

A number of studies support these findings and recommend
adapted forms of CBT for children with autism that take into
consideration their social communication deficits. Specifically, it
is suggested that CBT be delivered with special attention given to
nonverbal deficits and underdeveloped social skills. This is said
to be accomplished by:

◆ The use of visual supports to translate complex concepts
   into more concrete terms and to support emotional recognition and expression (e.g., feeling thermometers depicting ranges of emotions)
◆ Embedding emotional recognition and social skills
   instruction into traditional CBT sessions to compensate
   for these deficits and to support the processing of social
   situations and social problem solving

Cognitive Behavioral Intervention Strategies (CBIS)

The National Professional Development Center (NPDC) on
Autism Spectrum Disorder identified Cognitive Behavioral
Intervention Strategies (CBIS) as an evidence-based practice for
children with autism, regardless of whether or not they have co-
occurring mental health conditions. In 2014 and 2020, the NPDC

conducted a comprehensive review of studies evaluating CBIS with individuals with autism and reported the following:

♦ CBIS were effective for elementary school-aged children (6–11 years) to high school-aged youth (15–18 years)
♦ CBIS were used effectively to address social, communication, behavior, cognitive, adaptive, mental health, and academic outcomes
♦ CBIS can be used as part of an intervention package in combination with other identified evidence-based interventions for children and youth with autism

Quick Start to Using Cognitive Behavioral Therapy

There are a number of ways you can introduce cognitive behavioral approaches to help your child develop emotional and self-regulation skills:

♦ One, by participating in structured CBT therapeutic sessions with your child
♦ Two, by using CBIS in the home

Locate a Qualified Cognitive Behavioral Therapy Provider Near You

If your child is experiencing the level of distress that is described in the case study above, then seeking CBT from a trained and licensed professional will bring you and your child some welcomed relief. Be sure to choose a provider that:

♦ Specializes in CBT as opposed to traditional talk therapy
♦ Is trained and experienced in using the methods that make CBT impactful for children with autism (described above)
♦ Has knowledge and experience in working with children your child's age
♦ Has knowledge and experience in working with children with autism and any co-occurring conditions your child may have

- Incorporates parent coaching into sessions and provides "homework" to practice learned strategies in real life settings
- Develops a time-limited treatment plan with specific goals and identified intervention procedures—CBT is not meant to go on forever unless different goals or skills are being addressed over time
- Is a good financial fit- often, those who specialize in CBT and have expertise in autism do not take insurance or are "out of network providers" only. This will not always be the case, but it is common and we do not want this to be a surprise after you receive your first bill! Ask up front what the fee structure is, what insurance is accepted, and if there are any flexible payment plans if this is a constraint for your family

Use Cognitive Behavioral Intervention Strategies in the Home with the Whole Family

There are a number of ways you can use CBIS to teach relaxation and stress reduction strategies to your child and anyone else who can benefit in a concrete and positive way. Here are a few quick CBIS to try first to get started.

- **Social Narratives:** These are short and simple stories that visually depict social and emotional situations and calming behaviors using pictures and developmentally appropriate and reinforcing language. In book or virtual form, social narratives can be used to help your child label thoughts and emotions, recognize bodily cues connected to fear and anxiety, and follow multi-step calming routines. You can make these yourself using pictures of your child or you can download one from the internet. Check out this resource from the Indiana Institute on Disability and Community for some examples: https://www.iidc .indiana.edu/irca/articles/writing-and-using-social-narratives.html
- **Video Modeling:** Take a short video of you performing a calm down routine that can be used to help your child

practice the steps needed to do it on their own. If your child can perform the steps when calm, then it is better to record them doing it well so they can watch themselves later. In times of stress or anxiety, it is best to rely on visuals as much as possible and limit the amount of language used

◆ **Role Play**: Role play can be a great way to recreate challenging situations and provide opportunities for your child to practice responding differently in them. It is also a great way to prime your child before entering a situation that might be anxiety-provoking. You can model healthy responses in role play and reinforce your child's practice attempts

You can use one or all of these strategies. You can also use them with siblings and any other members of the family who may benefit. Be sure to introduce these strategies positively and proactively. When your child is already in an anxious state, this is not a teachable moment. Rather, healthy routines should be taught and practiced when you and your child are at your best. Once your child is more proficient at practicing these strategies, and has been consistently reinforced for doing so, then you can begin to use these visual strategies to prompt or redirect your child in naturally occurring situations.

Summary

Changing cognitive and behavioral patterns is not easy, but it can be done. Do not feel like you have to be your child's therapist. There is a reason why licensed professionals do what they do and do it well. Not only do they have specialized training and the benefit of a controlled clinical setting, they also have the objectivity needed to address mental health concerns in a systematic and neutral way. Rightfully so, they are not emotionally connected or drained by your child's distress. They are not feeling the guilt and frustration that parents often feel when they see their child struggling, but don't know how to help. So, let the therapists do their job, so you can continue doing the important work of caring for yourself and your child.

Be aware of your own unhealthy thinking patterns and tend to your own self-care routines. You too deserve relief and relaxation. Your whole family does. Choose a therapist wisely, be up front about what your family is struggling with, commit to any homework they assign, and trust the process. Use the strategies discussed here to model, teach, and reinforce the use of healthy relaxation and coping routines in the home. By doing so, you will provide your child and family with some relief now and also provide them with tools they can use in the future. Start today for a better tomorrow!

Resources

American Psychological Association: What is Cognitive Behavioral Therapy
https://www.apa.org/ptsd-guideline/patients-and-families/cognitive-behavioral
National Association of Cognitive Behavioral Therapists
https://www.nacbt.org/
The Autism Interaction Network: Cognitive Behavioral Therapy and Autism Spectrum Disorder
https://iancommunity.org/cs/simons_simplex_community/cognitive_behavioral_therapy

10

Toilet Training, Feeding, and Sleeping

Toilet Training, Feeding, and Sleeping Explained

The goal of every hard-working parent is to have a well-rested, well-fed, and contented child at the end of each day. It gives you a sense of relief and accomplishment. That is why toileting, feeding, and sleeping are often referred to as the "big three" in parenting books and blogs. These activities are the first and most cherished acts of care you give your child. They are also some of the more challenging hurdles you have to overcome in the journey of raising a healthy and independent child.

Here is what the "big three" have in common with each other:

♦ They are the most basic needs
♦ They happen every day
♦ The health of one impacts the others

Here is how the "big three" are different from child to child:

♦ Physical readiness will vary
♦ Nutritional and digestive health needs will vary
♦ Level of resistance/compliance will vary
♦ Household resources, schedules, and routines will vary

DOI: 10.4324/9781003285953-11

These self-care routines are exciting milestones when met, and sources of great anxiety and frustration when delayed. No matter how easy or how challenging the path, it is one that is deeply personal and emotional for you and your child. It may feel like you are breaking the bonds you so lovingly made with your child since birth, as you nudge them closer to doing self-care routines independently. You may also feel guilty, frustrated, and even jealous of others who are further along in this process at times. This is normal and expected, whether you are parenting a child with special needs or not.

You can anticipate some bumps in the road to self-care if you have not encountered them already. Here, we will provide you with what you need to know to overcome the challenges you may face when embarking on the journey towards independent self-care with your child.

What the Research Reports

Toileting, feeding, and sleep involve a number of factors including medical (health conditions), physical (gross motor, oral, digestive development), and behavioral (skill development and compliance). So, when trying to develop healthy toileting, feeding, and sleep routines all of these aspects of your child's health and well-being should be considered. You will likely have exhausted all of your "go-to" parenting resources and will benefit from understanding what the research says about supporting the "big three," while keeping the neurological aspects of autism in mind.

Toileting
In general, children with autism are toilet trained later than typically developing children and show more resistance to the process. It has been estimated that 59% of children with autism do not develop bladder or bowel control at 3.5 years of age, which is commonly achieved by healthy children around this time (Ledford & Gast, 2006; Keen et al., 2007). There are a number of reasons for this delayed milestone. First, their social communication

challenges may prevent them from communicating toileting needs and making sense of what is expected of them. They may not be able to imitate toileting behaviors observed in others. They may also lack the motivation to please caregivers by complying with newly introduced toileting routines.

Second, their difficulty processing sensory information and adapting to new sensory stimuli can result in heightened levels of anxiety, stress, and avoidant behaviors. For these reasons, it is understandable if you are hesitant and concerned about the impact toilet training will have on you and your child.

However, confusion about toilet training is not unique to parents of children with autism. Expectations for when and how toilet training should occur are greatly influenced by a number of factors including cultural expectations, familial expectations, and societal norms. One thing is for sure, there is no fixed time-table. In general, research indicates the following for typically developing and healthy children:

♦ In western cultures, the average toilet training age to begin is 24–36 months
♦ On average, bladder and bowel control is possible by 18 months of age
♦ Earlier toilet training may take longer
♦ Earlier toilet training is not known to cause psychological or behavioral problems
♦ Later toilet training is associated with increased risk for bladder problems

Note, that it is indeed a process, and one that may not be completed within a specified timeline or on a predictable trajectory. Overall there are two goals toilet training aims to accomplish:

1. The ability to recognize the need to use the toilet (physiological)
2. The ability to complete the sequence of steps required to use the toilet (behavioral)

Therefore, it is important to focus on child-specific signs of readiness to begin working towards these goals and consider where your child might need the most support. This includes assessing physical signs, behavioral signs, and prerequisite skills needed to communicate a need to use the toilet and to complete a healthy routine when using the toilet. Some examples are:

♦ Showing signs of bladder control by staying dry for longer periods of time
♦ Expressing interest in the toileting behaviors of others
♦ Showing signs of discomfort/attempts to remove wet or soiled diapers
♦ Communicating in some way when urination or defecation is occurring
♦ Gross motor control needed to sit upright, etc.
♦ Physical dexterity to remove clothes, etc.
♦ Ability to imitate actions of others
♦ Ability to communicate the need to use the toilet (verbally or nonverbally)
♦ Ability to respond to a request/direction (verbally or nonverbally)

There is no "one size fits all" approach for toilet training healthy children. Some favor parent-led methods and others favor more child-led methods. Both have some evidence of success and there are advantages and disadvantages to each. Some commonalities across successful approaches include:

♦ All adhere to health and safety guidelines (e.g., American Academy of Pediatrics)
♦ All encourage praise (e.g., positive verbal feedback)
♦ All incorporate positive reinforcement (e.g., small and incremental rewards)

Along with the general guidelines for typically developing children, there is research specific to toilet training your child with autism that can help you overcome your hesitancy. In 2010, Kroeger and Sorensen reviewed the literature focused on toilet training methods used with children with autism and other developmental disabilities and identified a number of effective strategies for decreasing the duration of time it takes for children with autism to achieve this milestone. Here, the authors highlighted:

◆ The use of urine/enuresis alarms, better known as "bedwetting alarms," to learn more about your child's elimination schedule and to prompt initiation of the toileting routine

◆ The adoption of more intensive training methods based on the Rapid Training Method (RTT) protocol described by Azrin and Foxx. This method involves increasing fluid intake, frequent parent-led trips to the toilet, and adhering to a systematic set of procedures for successes and accidents

In 2017, Francis, Mannion, and Leader reviewed studies published after the 2009 article described above and offered a number of additional strategies successfully used with children with autism including:

◆ Video modeling (depicting a model engaging in the targeted toileting behaviors)

◆ Visual schedules (pictures depicting each step in order)

◆ Scheduled chair sitting (seating the child in a chair next to the toilet in scheduled intervals)

◆ Communication training and visual aids (use of cue cards, visual communication methods, speech generating devices, etc.)

◆ Dry checks (scheduled checks during potty training trials)

◆ Positive reinforcement (praise for dryness during checks, etc.)

Feeding

Eating is one of the most sensory-rich experiences we partake in on a daily basis. Preparing and enjoying meals involves a number of textures, temperatures, aromas, and flavors. It is also a valued social experience as families and friends come together to share conversation and celebrate milestones, holidays, and cultural traditions. We understand you are not only concerned about nourishing your child's health. You also want to help them develop the skills, tolerance, and motivation needed to eat a variety of foods and be meaningfully included in mealtime routines and events. This is why there are a few overarching goals related to overcoming feeding issues:

1. To rule out medical issues that prevent safe and healthy eating
2. To expand the variety of foods your child eats and digests well
3. To increase safe and independent use of feeding materials
4. To teach and reinforce behaviors required to participate in mealtime routines

By two years of age, most children are able to tolerate or enjoy foods with a variety of textures and flavors. They may have preference for some food groups or flavors over others. However, their choices are not as restrictive as those observed in children with autism. By the age of two, children are also becoming more proficient at using forks, spoons, and cups with more independence. Children with autism may be more delayed in reaching these milestones and require more focused intervention. This is because feeding and eating span a number of developmental domains that are impacted by autism:

- ◆ Oral motor development
- ◆ Cognitive development
- ◆ Speech and language development
- ◆ Gross and fine motor development
- ◆ Behavioral development

It has been estimated that 46–75% of children with autism have feeding and mealtime challenges that cannot be dismissed as typical "picky eating" habits common to young children. Additionally, approximately 89% of children with autism exhibit challenging mealtime behaviors (Ledferd & Gast, 2007). Unlike typically developing children, these feeding and mealtime concerns presented by children with autism should not be "waited out." They will not be outgrown and they can lead to a number of health and behavioral issues that persist through adulthood. There are a number of professionals that can support your child's eating and mealtime challenges if needed:

- ◆ Occupational therapists
- ◆ Speech and language pathologists
- ◆ Physical therapists
- ◆ Behavioral therapists

Some children will have more complex medical needs that require more focused assessment and expert intervention such as:

- ◆ **Feeding disorders:** Warning signs include but are not limited to poor weight gain, bottle or feeding tube dependence, excessive pickiness or food refusal, excessive stress, anxiety, and/or tantrum meantime behaviors
- ◆ **Swallowing disorders:** Warning signs include but are not limited to excessive coughing, drooling, storing foods in cheeks, and frequent spitting-up or out of foods

If you observe any of the above in your child, seek help from expert professionals. Treatment for these disorders is available through in-patient and out-patient clinics. They can be treated by an interdisciplinary team of experts. For less complex challenges, research supports a number of techniques for increasing your child's tolerance for new foods and developing skills and motivation for participating in mealtime routines. Here we will highlight a few you can safely and comfortably try at home.

Desensitization

Desensitization is a process for building your child's tolerance for new foods. To understand desensitization, imagine yourself getting prepared to take a swim in a cold ocean on a rough day. Rather than jumping right in and swimming way out, you are more likely to stand and observe the waves, dip your toe in the water, wade in the shallow surf, and then slowly submerge yourself in the water and head further out negotiating one wave at a time. It is a slower process, but also a more enjoyable and safe one.

Desensitization in feeding involves exposing your child to less desired textures, tastes, smells are mealtime behaviors one step at a time, in a slow gradual manner over time. For example, you may want your child to start to eat yogurt. You might first just ask your child to smell it on a spoon, then touch the spoon to their lip, then lick the spoon and so on and so forth. This technique is paired with positive reinforcement. Compliance with each step is immediately followed with reinforcement (praise or access to more preferred foods or items).

This technique is also commonly paired with visual supports before and after each trial. Visual cues such as first-then boards can be used to communicate to your child that a loved food will immediately follow a less preferred food. It also communicates that one is contingent upon the other and will only be made available following compliance with your low-demand request.

This gradual and systematic approach is designed to minimize resistant and avoidant behaviors that commonly occur with food refusal. However, it is important to note that placing new expectations or demands on your child in the feeding process can also provoke new challenging behaviors that will need to be addressed along the way.

Food Chaining

Food chaining is a form of desensitization. It is considered by some to be a "child-friendly" tolerance-building approach that begins with the foods your child is familiar with and tolerant of and introduces new tastes, textures, and temperatures from there. The similar foods are used to create "food chains" by linking new foods you want to introduce to those your child already accepts or loves.

To do this you need to first make a list of foods your child loves. Note common attributes to the list of loved foods (flavor, texture, color, temperature, method of eating, etc.). For example, your child might love chicken nuggets, but only one brand, one shape, and served only at the perfect temperature. The flavor, texture, temperature, shape, and finger food aspects of the loved chicken nuggets are all great starting points. However, it is not realistic to serve one "just right" chicken nugget at every meal for your child.

Rather, you will use this as a starting point to introduce a similar food. You may introduce it intermittently between bites of the food you have linked it to. Or, you might incorporate the new flavor into an old one to mask the intensity of the flavor but also pair it with one your child already enjoys. Once a new flavor, texture, or shape is accepted then you can continue in this fashion with the goal of slowly expanding your child's tolerance and hopefully enjoyment of a variety of healthy foods while keeping them content with what they already enjoy.

Both of the techniques discussed here rely heavily on the consistent use of effective behavioral strategies (e.g., prompting and reinforcement). If you are not making strides in feeding new foods to your child or are dealing with challenging mealtimes behavior, then you can consult with a behavioral therapist that uses principles of applied behavior analysis to set up more systematic feeding and mealtime protocols for you in the home.

Sleep

We don't have to tell you how important sleep is, or how the lack of it affects how well we function on any given day. Chances are you are reading this chapter with the weariness only a hardworking and sleep-deprived parent can understand. If you and your child are not getting a good night's sleep, you are not alone. A 2019 study by Mazurek and colleagues, one of the largest studies conducted on the co-occurrence of autism and sleep disorders to date reported that up to 80% of preschool-aged children with autism have sleep issues. A number of studies confirm the frequency and intensity of sleep-related issues in children with autism and note that these issues can persist in adolescence and adulthood without focused intervention. Here, it was noted that when compared to typically developing children, children with autism have:

◆ More difficulty falling asleep
◆ Sleep for fewer hours each night

◆ Less time in the most restorative stage of sleep (Rapid Eye Movement [REM])
◆ Wake up more frequently throughout the night
◆ Have more frequent bedwetting issues

There are a number of theoretical explanations for the sleep disturbances observed in children with autism. Overall, research suggests that issues with sleep are closely correlated with the neurology of autism and commonly co-occurring conditions noting:

◆ Increased hyperactivity (difficulty winding down)
◆ Heightened sensory needs (increased sensitivity to light, sound, temperature)
◆ Heightened anxiety (separation and downtime challenging)
◆ Heightened digestive issues (abdominal discomfort, constipation)

According to the Mazurek study and supporting research, sleep deprivation has a detrimental effect on learning and behavior, as well the overall health and well-being of children and their caregivers. Research suggests that the following autism-related challenges are exasperated by sleep disturbances:

◆ Increased behavior problems
◆ Increased stereotypy and repetitive behaviors
◆ Increased sensory challenges
◆ Increased anxiety
◆ Increased inattention
◆ Increased hyperactivity
◆ Increased gastrointestinal issues

If you are wondering if this is a "chicken or the egg" type dilemma, you are not alone. It is hard to know which comes first, these problems or sleep problems. What we do know is that autism is neurological and affects the whole body, so it is best to look at sleep-related issues in a whole-body context.

Research suggests that the sleep issues observed in children with autism may be more frequent or intense, but they are not entirely different from those that occur in typically developing children (Lord, 2019). With this in mind, the following interventions are recommended and should occur simultaneously with one another:

Diet Modifications

If your child has a known food allergy, intolerance, or a digestive disorder of any kind then their eating patterns will greatly impact their sleep. It is essential to rule out any medical conditions that may exasperate sleep issues or seek expert guidance on how known issues can be addressed in relation to sleep. Even children without diagnosed allergies or digestive challenges are impacted by the type, portion, and timing of foods before bedtime.

As stated earlier, there is no one size fits all diet. So, modifications for your child's diet require closer assessment by you and consultation with your medical professionals. To better inform you and those who support you, consider keeping a journal of the meals your child eats and the sleep patterns they experience each day. This will help you note any correlated issues and make modifications accordingly.

Additionally, there are a number of natural supplements (e.g., melatonin) that research has shown to be safe and effective in addressing sleep-related issues in children with and without autism (see previous chapters). Be sure to discuss sleep concerns with your child's doctor and get their expert opinions on what medications or supplements might benefit your child based on their unique health profile.

Environmental Modifications

Our bodies have an internal clock that sets our sleep-wake cycle in a 24-hour period. Referred to as "circadian rhythms," this internal clock is influenced by a number of environmental factors. Put simply, there are sights, sounds, and temperatures that our body associates with daytime or nighttime. These cue our brains to communicate to our bodies when it is time to get up and get going and when it is time to wind down and prepare for sleep. To stay on a natural and consistent sleep-wake cycle, we need to keep these environmental cues as natural and consistent as possible.

In modern families, this is more challenging as our days often begin before sunrise and end long after. Also, we are a technology-dependent society and the artificial light transmitted from the electronics we use each day tell lies to our brain about what time it is and where our bodies should be in the re-occurring sleep-wake cycle. To counteract interference with a healthy sleep-wake cycle that works for you and your child, you may need to:

◆ Block out natural light with blackout curtains
◆ Remove electronics early in the day/evening
◆ Keep the room cooler at night than kept in the day
◆ Reduce daytime noise after dark, or use white noise to cover it up
◆ Keep daytime clothes separate from nighttime clothes
◆ Keep daytime scents separate from nighttime scents

Behavioral Modifications

Good sleep depends on good sleep hygiene, or bedtime routines that promote healthy sleep patterns. The need to teach good sleep hygiene to children with autism is often overlooked. In addition to the neurological complexities discussed here, children with autism may not learn how to follow healthy daily routines just from observation or repetition over time. Once sleep disturbances occur, they are not likely to go away without direct instruction on how to complete bedtime routines and consistent reinforcement for adhering to expected bedtime behaviors. In order to teach and reinforce good sleep hygiene, consider using the following evidence-based practices:

◆ **Visual schedules/checklists:** Create a visual schedule for "getting ready for bed tasks" (bath time, Pjs, book reading, tuck in, lights down, etc.). Complete the bedtime routine the same way every night. If that is too complex to start, create a visual checklist for what "ready for bed looks like" and help your child check them off when complete. Be sure to provide positive reinforcement/praise for adhering to expected behavior

◆ **"Bed-time pass":** This strategy, promoted by Boys Town Center for Behavioral Health, involves parents giving their child a card (small durable pass) that they can use one time a night after tuck-in. The pass can be used for any of the usual bedtime requests (extra hug, the forgotten story, or the request for a special stuffed animal, etc.), but only once. It is simple but effective when used consistently. It gets the parent in the habit of tucking in and walking out and eases the child into the habit of tolerating the "walk-out" before using the pass. Be sure to provide positive reinforcement/praise for adhering to parameters

Research suggests that even the most challenging sleep disorders can be addressed with the right help at the right time. However, if sleep issues are interfering with your child's ability to function on a daily basis or if there are safety issues that stem from your child's night waking or resistance to bedtime routines, then do not hesitate to reach out for help from the experts discussed in this book.

Quick Start to Toilet, Feeding, and Sleep Training

Toilet, feeding, and sleep training, oh my! At first, the weight of the responsibility of these issues may seem like too much at once. Our first advice is to start with the following:

◆ Rule out any medical concerns your child may not be able to express
◆ Avoid comparing your child to siblings or other children
◆ Do not set artificial deadlines such as a pending birthday or starting school to meet these developmental milestones
◆ Seek expert advice, avoid unsolicited advice from others who may not understand autism
◆ Expect setbacks and celebrate small successes

You can rest assured that the interconnectedness of these routines means that by addressing one, you are making headway in addressing the others. Relax for a moment to prepare yourself, and then proceed confidently with the following mindset.

Care for Your Whole Child First

- ◆ Rule out any digestive/bowel disorders, food allergies, etc.
- ◆ Assess overall nutrition, diet, and supplements needs
- ◆ Know side effects of any prescribed medicines
- ◆ Respect that changes in daily routines need to be well timed for your child and family

Meet Your Child Where They Are Now

- ◆ Consider what foods, activities, responses are most reinforcing for your child
- ◆ Consider what challenging behaviors might need to be addressed first
- ◆ Consider what prerequisite skills might need to be taught first
- ◆ Consider your child's most reliable or preferred mode of communication

Seek Help from the Experts

Review each of the previous chapters of this book. This resource provides must-know information about nutrition, medication, development, behavior, and the professionals who can support you in meeting developmental milestones. Read these chapters in the context of these goals, determine where you may need some help, flip through to see who the experts are and what you can expect from them.

Summary

Consider your child's unique health, physiology, behavior, and communication needs when determining when and how to make changes to daily self-care routines. Remember, caring for your whole child means focusing on best practices for the health and safety of your child first. Although you will likely need to adjust expectations and approaches to develop healthy self-care routines for your child with autism, there is no set timeline or one-size-fits-all approach for doing so.

No matter how effective an approach is described to be in the research, it is important for you to consider your child's unique needs and preferences, as well as your own cultural values, belief systems, and parenting style. Seek help when needed. Try not to compare your child to others or judge yourself too harshly. Feel good about the meals shared, the tuck-ins provided and the loving care you provide each day to keep your child feeling nourished, safe, and provided for.

Resources

American Academy of Pediatrics
https://www.aap.org/
Association for Science in Autism Treatment
https://asatonline.org/research-treatment/clinical-corner/toilet-training/
https://asatonline.org/research-treatment/clinical-corner/improving-food-selectivity/
https://asatonline.org/research-treatment/clinical-corner/regulating-sleep/

References

Francis, K., Mannion, A., & Leader, G. (2017). The assessment and treatment of toileting difficulties in individuals with autism spectrum disorder and other developmental disabilities. *Review Journal of Autism and Developmental Disorders, 4*(3), 190–204.

Kroeger, K., & Sorensen, R. (2010). A parent training model for toilet training children with autism. *Journal of Intellectual Disability Research, 54*(6), 556–567.

Ledford, J., & Gast, D. (2006). Feeding problems in children with autism spectrum disorders: A review. *Focus on Autism and Other Developmental Disabilities*, *21*(3), 153–166. https://doi.org/10.1177/108 83576060210030401.

Lord, C. (2019). Taking sleep difficulties seriously in children with neurodevelopmental disorders and ASD. *Pediatrics*, *143*(3). https://doi.org/10.1542/peds.2018-2629.

Mazurek, M. O., Dovgan, K., Neumeyer, A. M., & Malow, B. A. (2019). Course and predictors of sleep and co-occurring problems in children with autism spectrum disorder. *Journal of Autism and Developmental Disorders*, *49*(5), 2101–2115. https://doi.org/10.1007/s10803-019-03894-5.

11

Teacher Collaboration

Teacher Collaboration Explained

Communication with your child's teacher(s) is a vital part of your child's educational success. Think about this. Your elementary-age child will spend on average at least six hours a day for five days a week with the teacher. This equates to 30 hours per week. The average school year has 36 weeks per year. This equals 1,080 hours during the school year or 64,800 minutes. That is a lot of time. At the end of the school year, this teacher will know your child very well. Having a connection with your child's teacher is important and this develops over time.

Why wait until the open house or back to school night to connect with the teacher? Try to make the connection as soon as the school year starts. Set up a meeting as soon as you find out who your child's teacher is. Try to meet with the teacher either before the first day of school or within the first week of school.

If the teacher can't meet with you as soon as you want to, then write a letter to the teacher about your child. You can mail or email the letter to the teacher prior to your meeting. This shows you are reaching out to establish a connection.

Below is a sample letter that a parent wrote to her son's third grade teacher. She highlighted her son's strengths and potential areas of weakness. If appropriate for your child's education, you could write a letter like this:

DOI: 10.4324/9781003285953-12

Box 11.1 Sample Parent Letter

Dear Mrs. Petersen,

We look forward to working with you this year and, if needed, we are available to volunteer in the classroom. Last year Sammy had a very good year. These words describe some of Sammy's qualities: sensitive, likes to laugh, emotional, and routine-oriented.

Sammy has moderate autism and has been working with a board certified behavior analyist and licensed speech and language therapist for the past two years. He has made great progress and works hard to earn reinforcers. Sammy takes daily medication and at times his doctor might need your input about his school performance. He has an IEP and our main goal for Sammy is to continue to improve his communication. We find the following strategies work well with Sammy:

- Sammy is sensitive to loud noises so if you are aware there will be a fire drill, please take him outside before the alarm sounds
- A visual daily schedule helps him understand the day and anticipate transitions
- Encourage him to talk and respond to all his communication attempts
- When possible, seat him next to peers with good behavior
- Give him short sections of work and the opportunity to earn reinforcers
- Giving Sammy a helping job in the classroom boosts his confidence and he likes to help others

- In short, we believe you will enjoy having Sammy in your class and we look forward to working with you and assisting in any way possible. We believe open and frequent communication is very important.

Sincerely,
Mrs. Dolly R.

If your child is in middle or high school, teacher communication is just as important as in elementary school. However, many parents communicate less with teachers during these years. Avoid this pitfall. Yes, your child has more teachers but continue to write your letter to teachers. Continue to meet with the teachers. Middle and high school teachers usually meet as a team so you might address all teachers together rather than individually. However, if there is a class that is particularly challenging for your child then schedule an individual meeting with that teacher at a later time.

This is how one parent described the importance of communication:

> At our annual IEP for my 14-year-old son who is on the autism spectrum, I typically have a good experience for a number of reasons. Most importantly, I have a good relationship with his teacher. She keeps me well informed on a daily if not weekly basis on his progress. If for some reason, I have not kept in touch, I make a point of doing so. Also, I am well aware of his goals for speech, occupational therapy and his educational curriculum. This way I can keep on top of his progress.
>
> If there is ever a question about how a goal is being implemented, I ask immediately. I feel open lines of communication are the most important when working with the staff to prepare the most complete IEP for my son. I also always try to incorporate more generalized goals for my son that may not be a part of a special needs program. I think it is important to incorporate art, music, science and social studies into his IEP goals. I suggested that he know capitols of cities for instance, create art projects to allow him to expand his educational experience, or to learn to use email. Everyone must have extra-curricular activities and my child works so hard daily that he needs other outlets to express himself. Who knows what talents lie within unless we try to tap into them?

122 ◆ Teacher Collaboration

This parent understood that the connection and communication with teachers benefited her son. If you want your child to excel and learn during the school year communicate with the teacher. This will create a connection. Think about this. Will your child work better and learn more with a teacher that cares about him? You know the answer is, "absolutely." If you communicate with the teacher, they will get to know your child as an individual and start to develop deeper care and concern for them.

In Chapter 12 we discussed that it is helpful to maintain organized records. You might keep a notebook to document contact with your child's teacher using the sample format below. Many parents keep electronic notes on their smart device. Maintaining records is helpful should a need arise.

Teacher/Administrator Contact Sheet

Date: _____

Time: _____

Person(s) Communicated with:

Summary of Conversation/Meeting/Contact:

What the Research Reports

Most parents value a strong parent-teacher partnership. Researchers Syriopoulous-Delli, Cassimos, and Polychrnopoulous (2016) studied teacher and parent collaboration by surveying 171 teachers and 50 parents of children with autism. Both groups rated the communication and collaboration between teachers and parents as critically important with 96.5% of teachers in agreement and 100% of parents in agreement. While life is busy, making time to know your child's teacher is one key element in your child's success.

Houser and colleagues (2015) investigated parents' perceptions regarding parent and teacher collaboration and identified three common themes. First, the majority of parents reported having a positive relationship with their child's special education school personnel. Second, an advantage of home-school communication was parents knew how their child was progressing and what they could do at home to support school learning. Third, many parents noted their child's special education teacher was not properly trained to work with children with autism.

Effective problem solving is an important part of parent and teacher collaboration. Azad and colleagues (2016) studied this and positively noted, "Both parents and teachers reported using interventions for children with ASD and were observed to communicate about using specific intervention strategies" (p. 10). They found that teachers did most of the problem solving by discussing data, intervention plans, and students' strengths.

Of course, no relationship is completely perfect and problems can exist within the teacher-parent collaboration process. Tucker and Schwartz (2013) surveyed 135 parents and encouragingly stated parents reported high levels of involvement in their child's education. Parents' main concerns were when:

◆ Parents' ideas and suggestions were not valued
◆ There was no regular communication
◆ The IEP was created without parent input
◆ Outside provider input was not considered

Parents felt valued when:

◆ They participated in writing IEP goals
◆ They provided input into the curriculum and instructional approaches
◆ Had a voice in selecting their child's placement options
◆ Outside provider information was considered

Jan Blancher, Ph.D., is a professor and director of the Support, Education, Advocacy, Resources, Community, Hope (SEARCH) Family Autism Resource Center at the University of California

Riverside. Currently she is studying factors that contribute to positive school experiences for children with autism and preliminary research from her center identified one key factor is having a positive student–teacher relationship. This has implications for parents because while, at times, we might disagree with educators, it is still important to maintain a positive relationship for your child's sake. The last thing you want is for your child's teacher to treat your child poorly because of a parent–teacher problem. Your good relationship will likely lay the groundwork for your child to develop a good relationship with the teacher.

Quick Start to Teacher Collaboration

Knowing that parent-teacher collaboration is important, reflect upon the relationship between you and your child's teacher(s). You can take the next steps to strengthen the relationship as well as let the teacher know you appreciate her or him. There is not a one-size-fits-all approach to building strong relationships and collaboration with teachers takes work. Some key ingredients for success include:

- ◆ Sharing pertinent information
- ◆ Establishing the right communication tool
- ◆ Maintaining honesty and openness
- ◆ Communicating intentionally
- ◆ Being interactive
- ◆ Maintaining the human touch

Some parents (and teachers) are better communicators than others. It can be helpful to have a communication schedule that includes the frequency of expected communications and process by which you'll communicate. Don't be afraid to directly ask the teacher, "How do you prefer to be communicated with?" Your child's teacher might be more available Monday through Thursday after school as compared to Friday or over the weekend. If you know your child's teacher's preferred communication method and times she is available, then you won't worry if she does not reply to your text after 5pm. You'd expect a reply the next morning.

Dr. Toby Honsberger is the Els Center for Excellence Learning Academy Executive Director and has supported hundreds of teachers and parents. He shares,

> As with any good collaboration, communication is key and quality collaboration consists of two-way communication. Parents often request regular communication from teachers to learn how a student's day was or what is being worked on. In addition, parents also provide teachers with valuable information to improve the education of their son or daughter. Providing general information such as likes and dislikes, skills, and challenges, and/or past successful or unsuccessful instructional strategies can help a teacher establish an effective educational plan for a student. Information about family members, what the family did on the weekend, what was for breakfast etc. can be valuable information to facilitate social communication at school. Daily communication about how they slept, how the morning went, and/or how they are feeling can prepare a teacher for daily expectations.

When school and home needs are on the same page, your child's likelihood for success increases. Some teachers use:

- ◆ Newsletters
- ◆ A communication log
- ◆ IEP updates
- ◆ Your child's completed work
- ◆ Report cards and progress reports
- ◆ Class Dojo
- ◆ Email
- ◆ Texts
- ◆ Conferences in person, or via Zoom, FaceTime, Skype™

Teachers are often overworked and underappreciated. You might show your teacher appreciation by:

- ◆ Writing a complimentary note
- ◆ Volunteering in the classroom
- ◆ Donating materials such as copy paper or disinfecting wipes
- ◆ Becoming a class sponsor (if the school offers this)
- ◆ Telling the administrator how much you appreciate the teacher
- ◆ Providing a holiday gift
- ◆ Donating food for a class celebration
- ◆ Helping set up a Donors Choose campaign for class materials

Teachers in middle and high school appreciate your help as well and often get overlooked since most parent involvement is in elementary.

Summary

Your child's teacher is a key variable in your child's learning and it's likely you and the teacher will value communication. Work together to determine each other's preferred communication method. Help the teacher understand your child's preferences, personality, and pickiness. The teacher wants to know from you what works at home so she can follow through in the classroom just as you want to know how to support classroom instruction at home. While there can be disagreements, amicably solving these benefits your child. Appreciate teachers (and therapists) with random acts of kindness. What is your next step?

Resources

Class Dojo
https://www.classdojo.com

Donors Choose
https://www.donorschoose.org
Teachers Pay Teachers Autism Helper Home School Communication Packet
https://www.teacherspayteachers.com/Product/Home-School-Communication-Packet-1414380
SEARCH Family Autism Research Center
https://searchcenter.ucr.edu

References

Azad, G. F., Kim, M., Marcus, S. C., Mandell, D. S., & Sheridan, S. M. (2016). Parent-teacher communication about children with autism spectrum disorder: An examination of collaborative problem-solving. *Psychology in the Schools, 53*(10), 1071–1084. https://doi.org/10.1002/pits.21976.

Houser, M. A., Fontenot, C. L., & Spoede, J. (2015). Home-school collaboration for students with ASDs: Parents' perspectives. *Journal of the American Academy of Special Education Professionals, 83*, 97.

Syriopoulou-Delli, C. K., Cassimos, D. C., & Polychronopoulou, S. A. (2016). Collaboration between teachers and parents of children with ASD on issues of education. *Research in Developmental Disabilities, 55*, 330–345. https://doi.org/10.1016/j.ridd.2016.04.011.

Tucker, V., & Schwartz, I. (2013). Parents' perspectives of collaboration with school professionals: Barriers and facilitators to successful partnerships in planning for students with ASD. *School Mental Health, 5*(1), 3–14. https://doi.org/10.1007/s12310-012-9102-0.

12

Effective IEPs and IFSPs

Effective Individual Education Programs (IEPs) and Individual Family Support Plans (IFSPs) Explained

When your child is diagnosed with autism, he or she might be eligible to receive special education services via the federal law called the Individuals with Disabilities Education Act, which is often referred to using the acronym IDEA. We say your child "might" be eligible as just because a child has an autism diagnosis, a diagnosis alone does not automatically equate to eligible for services as your child must show a "need" for support and services. School district personnel document the need for supports and services in various ways such as using behavioral observations, rating scales, testing, communication, and activities of daily living such as your child's ability to understand safety.

The IDEA specifies that all school-aged children (ages 3–21) with disabilities are entitled to a "Free Appropriate Public Education (FAPE)." This means your child can receive educational services, speech and language, occupational or physical therapy, behavioral support, special transportation, and more. Your child's services are decided by a team of professionals and *you*. This group is often called the Individualized Education Program (IEP) team.

The collaborative group works together to discuss and write your child's IEP. The IEP is often referred to as the blueprint for your child's education because once written, it specifies all

DOI: 10.4324/9781003285953-13

services and supports your child will receive. You must sign and give parental consent for the school staff to evaluate your child and to start providing services.

Your child's IEP is revised at least once a year and you may schedule a review meeting at any time. The required components of an IEP include:

- Present levels of academic achievement and functional performance
- Measurable annual goals
- A process for measuring of progress toward the annual goals
- Statements related to special education, related services, supplementary aids, and services based on peer-reviewed research to the extent practical and program modification or supports for school personnel
- An explanation of the extent, if any, to which the child will not participate with nondisabled children
- Appropriate accommodations that are necessary to measure academic achievement and functional performance of the child on state and district-wide assessments as well as a statement of any needed alternative assessments on a particular state or district-wide assessment
- The projected date for the beginning of services and modification, the anticipated frequency, location, and duration of these services and any modifications
- A statement that by age 16 measurable postsecondary goals, based on age-appropriate transition assessments, are developed. These are related to training, education, employment, and, where appropriate, independent living skills and transition services needed to help the child to reach goals. There must be a statement related to transfer of rights no later than one year before child reaches age of majority

If your child is age birth through age three, a different plan is written called the Individual Family Support Plan or IFSP. This plan also specifies the services that your child and *you* will receive. Professionals recognize that a young child is part of a family system and therefore to help your child, professionals might need to help you as well. This could be providing you with information about government programs or access to respite care so you can have time to focus on your needs.

Your child's IFSP is revised once a year and reviewed at least every six months. The required components of an IFSP include:

◆ A statement of the infant or toddler with a disability's present levels of physical development (including vision, hearing, and health status), cognitive development, communication development, social or emotional development, and adaptive development

◆ A statement of the family's resources, priorities, and concerns related to enhancing the development of the child

◆ A statement of the measurable results or measurable outcomes expected to be achieved for the child (including pre-literacy and language skills, as developmentally appropriate for the child) and family, and the criteria, procedures, and timelines used to determine progress and if any revisions are needed

◆ A statement of the specific early intervention services necessary to meet the unique needs of the child and the family

◆ The length, duration, frequency, intensity, and method of delivering the early intervention services in the natural environment

◆ Identify medical and other services that the child or family needs or is receiving through other sources

◆ The name of the service coordinator from the profession most relevant to the child's or family's needs who will be responsible for implementing the early intervention services identified in a child's IFSP

◆ The steps and services to be taken to support the smooth transition of the child to preschool services

Preparing in advance for the IEP or IFSP meeting can help you advocate for your child's education. Thus, strive to become a lifelong learner about your child's disability and how it affects him or her. You can think about and write down the most important skills you would like your child to learn. Research the benefits of specific therapies such as speech or occupational therapy and, if appropriate, be prepared to discuss why you believe these might help your child. Come prepared with a list of questions to ask at the meeting and we provided some questions you might ask in the "Quick Start to IEPs" section below.

Remember, you understand and know your child best and you are your child's best advocate!

What the Research Reports

Within the IDEA, the acronym IEP stands for an Individualized Education Program and this federal law discusses the IEP in Section 1414 (d) (1). You can locate the full description via an internet search for "IDEA section 1414 (d) (1)" or by searching "Office of Special Education Programs." The IEP becomes a binding contract between you and the school district.

The quality of IEPs varies by state, school district, and even individual school. Ruble and colleagues (2010) conducted a study to examine IEPs of 35 children with autism across school districts in two states and found most IEPs were lacking. They noted, "Measurability of IEP objectives appeared to be one of the greatest areas of need. In particular, specified criteria for goal measurement and success were lacking" (p. 8).

In a 2013 study, Ruble and McGrew studied factors leading to better IEP goal attainment for children with autism. They examined four factors (child, teacher, intervention practice, and implementation practice) and reported IEP quality and child engagement were the largest contributing factors for obtaining IEP goals. This implied that if you want your child to obtain his or her IEP goals, you must start with a well written IEP and then have your child engaged in intervention instruction.

These studies support that a well written, quality IEP with measurable goals is an important part of the equation for helping your child. The IEP meeting can be intimidating for parents and Fish (2006) investigated an autism group's experiences at IEP meetings. The Texas families reported parents perceived being treated more positively with the presence of an advocate at their IEP meetings. When parents were asked what other parents could do to improve IEP meetings they indicated: becoming knowledgeable about special education issues, being involved in the IEP meeting and creating a cooperative atmosphere, and becoming knowledgeable about special education law in order to advocate for services.

The takeaway points from research are:

◆ Your child's IEP is important
◆ You want the IEP to have measurable goals and objectives
◆ When possible, bring an advocate to IEP meetings
◆ If your child is engaged in learning, he has the best opportunity to achieve his IEP goals

Since it is important to have measurable IEP goals, some educators and parents use the SMART acronym to help remember key components for writing measurable IEP goals. Hedin and DeSpain (2018) described SMART as:

◆ Specific
◆ Measurable
◆ Action verbs
◆ Realistic
◆ Time limited

As a parent, it is not your responsibility to write IEP goals as that requirement falls upon educators. However, it is important to be able to recognize the SMART components to know if your child's IEP goals are written well. The following are examples of SMART IEP goals:

◆ Given a first-grade addition math computation paper and pencil and a verbal prompt to work for 3 minutes, Erin will solve and write the answers with at least 10 problems correct in three consecutive trials by November 1

◆ When provided the appropriate materials (e.g., soap, sink, towel) and verbally prompted to wash hands, Colin will wash hands before eating or after returning to the classroom from specials, completing four of five steps independently, five days per week for two consecutive weeks by end of the quarter

◆ Given an adult's verbal prompt, Mario will provide a yes or no response to need to use the toilet through verbal, gestures, or pictorial supports for three prompts per day over five days by March 31

Many of the principles for having an effective IEP also relate to you receiving an effective IFSP. Xu (2008) reported "A key to effective IFSPs is including outcomes that address the entire family's well-being and not only outcomes designed to benefit the child's development" (p. 3). IFSPs written with this in mind tend to be more effective than those focusing only on the child's development.

If you are the parent of a young child with autism, you might be investigating which program is best for your child. Myers and Johnson (2007) summarize that effective early childhood intervention for children with ASDs should include the following components:

◆ Provide early intervention as soon as an ASD diagnosis is considered

◆ Intensive teaching for at least 25 hours a week, 12 months a year

◆ Low student-to-teacher ratios using 1:1 instruction and small group instruction

◆ Include the family

◆ Interaction with typically developing peers

◆ Measure and document the child's progress and adjust programming when needed

◆ Provide predictable routine, visual activity schedules, and clear physical boundaries to minimize distractions

◆ Include strategies for generalization and maintenance of new skills

◆ Use curricula that include communication, social skills, functional skills, using strategies to reduce behaviors, teaching cognitive skills, and readiness and academic skills

These principles can be reframed into questions you can ask potential schools for your child:

◆ What is your teacher-to-student ratio?
◆ How is the family included in your program?
◆ Do you have students without disabilities in the class?
◆ How do you report progress to parents?
◆ What is a typical daily schedule and how does my child understand the schedule?
◆ What curriculum do teachers use?

Your involvement in making decisions about your child's education will position your child to obtain the best outcomes.

Quick Start to IEPs

Most children with autism have IEPs (ages 3–21) so the remainder of this section will describe IEP processes.

Daniely lins da Silva, a parent of a teen son, offers this advice, "Get familiar with how IEPs and special education work so you can better advocate for your child. And get connected with others to find support because it truly does take a village." Since the IEP is the blueprint for your child's education, then it is helpful to understand who exactly designs the IEP. The design team members are the individuals comprising the IEP team and include:

◆ You
◆ Your child's special education teacher or a service provider
◆ A school district representative qualified to supervise special education instruction and is knowledgeable about district resources
◆ A person qualified to interpret testing results

- ◆ One or more of your child's general education teachers
- ◆ Others who have knowledge or expertise about your child such as speech-language or other therapists
- ◆ Your child, if appropriate

Others who are not required members, but might attend your child's IEP meeting, include:

- ◆ Advocates
- ◆ Medical professionals
- ◆ Family
- ◆ An attorney
- ◆ Transition specialists,
- ◆ Other school system representatives

We've participated in IEP meetings and realize this process can be somewhat intimidating because there are usually five or more professionals attending and often just one little bitty you. Therefore, we believe it is helpful to have another person attend the meeting with you. This could be your spouse, significant other, family member, friend, retired teacher, or other advocate. The person does not necessarily have to be an expert in the special education process as sometimes it's helpful for moral support and to have another set of ears to listen and make notes.

Our personal experience is that most dads or male family figures do not attend IFSP or IEP meetings. However, a male caregiver's perspective and input is important. Therefore, when a dad or other male attends the meeting it makes a strong statement and can show a united front. Although certainly not required, we encourage you to bring your child's father to the meeting with you.

Life is busy so it is understandable if you can't bring another person with you. So think about the message you convey when you show up to your child's IEP meeting on time, nicely dressed, with a 4-inch 3-ring binder organized with all your child's paperwork, and a list of questions you are ready to ask. The school staff quickly get the message that you mean business.

Consider taking these questions with you and asking them until you get a straightforward answer. Lay it all on the line because if you don't advocate for your child, who will?

1. Is this the best you can do for my child?
2. Are the annual goals SMART goals?
3. How will you document, over time, that my child makes progress?
4. What is the best available evidenced-based (reading, math, language, social skills, etc.) practice to help my child?
5. What technology is available to help my child?
6. Does the special education teacher hold a teaching degree in special education?
7. Are the services made up if the teacher or therapist is absent?
8. Can my child be held back?
9. Who receives a copy of the IEP?
10. What do I do if I want to change the IEP later?

Below we provide insider information from a retired ESE director to offer you pertinent information regarding the IEP process.

Box 12.1 A Former ESE Director's Tips for Getting a Great IEP

By Cathleen Blair

Many times parents come into a meeting for their child and become intimidated by the number of people around the table and become silent. Remember, this meeting is about your child. You know your child far better than anyone sitting in the room. Don't be afraid to ask questions or for clarification if you don't understand what someone has said. As educators, we want to help you understand and participate in the IEP process so that we can all work together to help your child. To get a great IEP for your child:

- Spend some time the night before the meeting writing down pertinent information about your child. This helps us because your input is valuable as well as required
- Respect the perspectives of all the attendees as they too should respect your opinion
- Be aware that the schools may have limitations so be creative. Sometimes some of the best solutions don't need to be expensive
- Stay on topic during the meeting. Don't bring up what happened in kindergarten when you are working with your child in the fifth grade
- Watch your nonverbal language too. If you fold your arms or sigh you might be giving off an impression that you are angry. Request a break if you feel frustrated and ask to speak with the person in charge of the IEP meeting
- Remember, an IEP must include the special services and accommodations that are necessary to enable the child to participate and progress in the general curriculum. That is not the same as including the entire educational curriculum itself
- Every child is required to meet standards set by the state. These standards are available to parents from the internet or from the teacher. What the IEP should indicate is what accommodations need to be made or what additional services should be given so that child can meet those standards. This could mean, for example, that a student needs to pass Algebra but because of the disability, the student will first learn fractions, then algebraic formulas, then complete the first semester in year one and in year two, and then progress to figuring out four step algebra equations
- Some parents want every step written on an IEP - like a contract - something that's not required or necessary
- Remember, your child's IEP will help the teachers and yourself show the way, a year at a time, to the ultimate

goal of graduation and employment. If everyone remembers that the IEP can guide and improve your child's education by identifying his needs based on current performance, provide the necessary services to address those needs, and objectively measure progress towards the goal

Organize Your Records

Preparation is key to success in most endeavors. The volume of paperwork in special education can be overwhelming. Each IEP is usually 5–10 pages and it is rewritten every year. In addition to your child's IEPs, you also have testing reports on your child. Then there are report cards and any yearly testing from the school. When you think about this, it is a lot of papers to keep track of. You need a system to organize your records or they become a huge, messy, unorganized file folder of documents.

We recommend scanning your documents and keeping them in electronic folders using the sections below. Other parents like the paper copies so they can bring them to the meeting or share them with new therapists as needed. In this case, it is helpful to purchase a three-ring notebook and divider tabs. Include the following sections: *IEP Documentation, Teacher Contacts, Administrator Contacts, Work Samples, Testing Records,* and *Report Cards.*

In the section labeled *IEP Documentation,* place all copies of your child's IEPs from current to oldest. Also include any of the procedural safeguard information, consent forms, and/or other official school district forms. This section is for any form you receive from the school district.

The second section is for all *Teacher Contacts* with your child's teacher(s). Use our sample form or create your own to document anytime you have contact with a teacher. If you have an email, print it out and place it in this section. Again, use the format of placing your most recent document in the front to oldest in the back of the section.

Administrator Contacts is the section for placing all communication with the school principal or assistant principal, Special Education Director, or any district staff member. You can use our form to document administrator contacts. It is important to document the person's name, date, and a brief summary of the communication. Again, print any email documentation and place it in order from most to least current.

Keep a section called *Work Samples* which includes representative work from your child. One way to think about what to place in this section is to use the IEP as a guide. Every IEP has annual goals and each annual goal represents a specific area of need (math, reading, written language, behavior, etc.). Select a representative piece of work for each annual goal area for each marking period in an academic year. That way you'll see progress and continuity as your child progresses throughout the year.

Testing Records includes any of the state- or school-wide testing results. In each state this type of test has a different name but measures the student's learning. For example, in Florida our test is called the Florida Standards Assessment. Children that do not take this test take an alternative assessment such as the Brigance. It is helpful to keep these records to show your child's progress across time.

The final notebook section is *Report Cards*. File the final report card for each year in this section since it has the grades from each marking period on it. If your child's final report card is not a cumulative report card with all previous grades on it then you may want to file each marking term report card.

By being proactive and organizing your child's paperwork, you have a system for keeping track of things. This system will be valuable if you ever run into problems with your child's school or in the event of mediation or any other arbitration process.

IEP Goals

There is no limit to the number of annual goals written on your child's IEP. If a skill is important to you or any IEP team member, it can become a goal. Anyone on the IEP team can suggest goals for your child. The IEP goals:

- Are decided by the IEP team
- Are for one year
- Should be measurable
- Document the important skills for your child to learn
- Can be academic, behavioral, daily living, speech or language, physical, emotional, etc.
- Are reported on each time a report is sent home
- Can be reviewed or revised at any time

Your child's IEP goals are based on what is most important for your child to learn and educators call this the "priority educational need." As you prepare for your child's IEP meeting, think and make notes on what you believe is most important for your child to learn. You can be specific and state you want your child to learn 20 more words to help with communication or to learn how to appropriately greet friends. IEP goals can include anything from toileting to graduating. The IEP team will use your input and write the SMART IEP goals for teachers or therapists to work on.

Placement and Services

The IEP specifies the type of program or class placement where your child will receive special education services. We want your child to be taught in what the IDEA calls the "least restrictive environment" or as close to typical as possible. The concept of least restrictive environment includes where your child spends time in school and how special education is provided. The IDEA requires:

- Your child receives education with peers without disabilities to the maximum extent possible
- Your child should not be removed from the general education classroom unless learning cannot occur even with supports of supplementary aids and services

Your child's individual needs and the IEP team consider your child's least restrictive environment placement. Since autism occurs from mild to severe, there is no one size fits all placement. Ideally, you want your child to be educated as close to home as possible and in the school he would attend if he did not have autism. Consider where your child might benefit the most from his education. The range of placements for all kids with disabilities from least restrictive to most restrictive include:

♦ General education classroom
♦ General education classroom with pull out resource room support
♦ General education classroom with part-time special education classroom
♦ Special education classroom, full time
♦ Special school
♦ Homebound
♦ Hospital or residential facility

There are pros and cons to each placement and you do not have to make the decision alone. Work with your child's IEP team, ask other parents of kids like yours, and do your own online research. If the IEP team is considering your child moving to a new school or class, request an in-person visit prior to agreeing. A firsthand visit is usually helpful to get a feel for the school, see the other children, and talk with teachers. Regardless of what educators say, an in-person visit prior to you signing is your right.

The IEP Annual Review

At the annual review you get a chance to review your child's progress. During this time you want to look at each annual goal and determine if your child achieved the goal. After all, the annual goal is based on the most important need your child has. This would be a great time to break out your well organized portfolio that includes work samples matched to annual goals. Making decisions for next year based on actual data is much more efficient than guessing or relying on memory.

If your child did not meet the annual goal ask questions. Don't assign blame. Ask questions such as, "What do you believe stopped my child from achieving the goal? How frequent was the instruction? (what you are asking here is was adequate time spent working on this goal or does the teacher believe he needs more time to master the skill) Was the way it was taught effective for my child? What might be changed to help my child meet this goal?"

Ask yourself, "Is this goal is still one of the most important needs for your child?" If you or the teacher suggests the goal should be carried over to the new IEP, ask yourself the question, "What will be different next year?" Is there a new instructional approach, more time spent on mastery, a new teacher, therapist, setting, or other critical factor for success? If there is not a critical change in how this goal is achieved, consider dropping it. For example, one parent explained, "The teachers kept on trying to get Michael to tie his shoes. For some reason his fingers just could not hold the laces the right way and it frustrated him. He would shut down and cry. They worked on this for two years without him mastering it. Finally, I insisted on just using Velcro straps."

Summary

As a parent of a child with autism, you are a required member of the IEP team and you get to choose your level of participation. You can be passive or active. We believe being an active participant helps you get the best IEP for your child. You understand your child best and can describe your child at a personal level to help the other team members' understanding. During the IEP meeting, you tell the team the most important skills you want your child to learn. These are written into IEP goals that he and his teachers will work on for a year. Key takeaway points include:

- When possible, bring another person or an advocate to the IEP meeting
- Create a system to keep your records organized
- Your child's IEP goals are based on the most important skills you want your child to learn
- When report cards come home you should get an update on your child's progress toward meeting the IEP annual goals
- At any time during the year, you can request an IEP review meeting

Resources

U.S. Department of Education IDEA website
https://sites.ed.gov/idea/
Understood.org
https://www.understood.org/articles/en/ifsp-what-it-is-and
-how-it-works
Wrightslaw.com
https://www.wrightslaw.com/info/iep.index.htm
Early Intervention Parent Leadership Project
https://eiplp.org/individualized-family-service-plan-ifsp/

References

Fish, W. W. (2006). Perceptions of parents of students with autism towards the IEP meeting: A case study of one family support group chapter. *Education*, *127*(1), 56–68.

Hedin, L., & DeSpain, S. (2018). SMART or not? Writing specific, measurable IEP goals. *Teaching Exceptional Children*, *51*(2), 100–110. https://doi.org/10.1177/0040059918802587.

Myers, S. M., Johnson, C. P., & American Academy of Pediatrics Council on Children with Disabilities. (2007). Management of children with autism spectrum disorders. *Pediatrics*, *120*(5), 1162–1182.

Ruble, L. A., McGrew, J., Dalrymple, N., & Jung, L. A. (2010). Examining the quality of IEPs for young children with autism. *Journal of Autism and Developmental Disorders*, *40*(12), 1459–1470. https://doi.org/10.1007/s10803-010-1003-1.

Ruble, L., & McGrew, J. H. (2013). Teacher and child predictors of achieving IEP goals of children with autism. *Journal of Autism and Developmental Disorders*, *43*(12), 2748–2763. https://doi.org/10.1007/s10803-013-1884-x.

Xu, Y. (2008). Developing meaningful IFSP outcomes through a family-centered approach using the double ABCX mod. *Young Exceptional Children*, *12*(1), 2–19. https://doi.org/10.1177/1096250608323993.

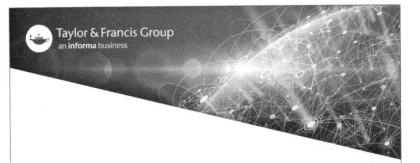

CPSIA information can be obtained
at www.ICGtesting.com
Printed in the USA
LVHW022331280822
727054LV00002B/240